# Fever Hospitals and Fever Nurses

'Margaret Currie has produced an excellent study of a much neglected subject... in a highly readable and rigorously researched way. Dr Currie has done us a great service by reminding us of the relevance of fever nursing to contemporary debates in nursing. I commend her book to you.' *Professor Anne Marie Rafferty, Dean and Chair in Nursing Policy at the Florence Nightingale School of Nursing and Midwifery, King's College, London*

This book is the first in-depth account of the development of fever hospitals and fever nursing – mainly in nineteenth and twentieth-century Britain. Rare social aspects are provided through probationers' views of their training and patient impact case studies, and key nurse leaders are featured, including ex-fever nurse Edith Cavell. *Fever Hospitals and Fever Nurses* provides new insights into how the predominantly female work force coped with epidemics, some of which were of national significance. The book also reflects current concerns, including the challenging nature of infectious disease and biological warfare.

*Fever Hospitals and Fever Nurses* will be vital reading for academics and students in nursing history and of great interest to current and former medical and nursing staff. Patients and their relatives, medical, social and family historians, students of women's history and control of infection nurses will all discover relevant data.

**Margaret Currie**, a registered general nurse, nurse tutor, and recently a senior lecturer at the University of Luton, has carried out extensive research into fever hospitals and fever nursing, and lectured on the subject in Britain and Canada. Her publications include articles on fever and small-pox nursing and she is a contributor to the *Dictionary of National Biography* (2004). She is currently Health Care Historian at the Luton and Dunstable Hospital NHS Trust and a Senior Research Fellow (Hon) at the University of Luton. Margaret is also a committee member of the Royal College of Nursing History of Nursing Society and she chairs the London and South East Group.

For
James, William, Edward, Victoria,
Emily, Oliver and Dominic

# Fever Hospitals and Fever Nurses

A British social history of fever nursing: a national service

**Margaret R Currie**

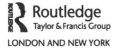
Routledge
Taylor & Francis Group

LONDON AND NEW YORK

First published 2005
by Routledge
2 Park Square, Milton Park, Abingdon, Oxon OX14 4RN

Simultaneously published in the USA and Canada
by Routledge

711 Third Avenue, New York, NY 10017

*Routledge is an imprint of the Taylor & Francis Group*

Transferred to Digital Printing 2005

First issued in paperback 2012

Typeset in 10/12 Baskerville by Scribe Design, Ashford, Kent

*British Library Cataloguing in Publication Data*
A catalogue record for this book is available from the British
Library

*Library of Congress Cataloging in Publication Data*
A catalog record for this book has been requested

ISBN 13: 978-0-415-64776-2 (pbk)
ISBN 13: 978-0-415-35164-5 (hbk)

# Contents

# Illustrations

**Figures**

## Tables

# Foreword

Margaret Currie has pulled off an impressive feat in producing this book. Not only has she produced an excellent study of a much neglected subject but she has accomplished this in a highly readable and rigorously - researched way. Dr Currie is to be congratulated on her foresight, tenacity and talent in writing this book. She has approached her subject from a variety of vantage points and, in the process, deployed different methods. This study is an exemplar of what a multi-method approach to historical writing and research can be. Blending survey data with oral history, biographical case studies as well as the more conventional documentary analysis, this study casts rare shafts of light into the lives of nurses, their careers as well as the settings in which patients were cared for. Furthermore, Margaret reminds us that fever nursing was not only about care but cure, at a time when therapies were rudimentary or involved little beyond reassurance.

I am delighted to see this book appear in print; not only because my mother features as one of the subjects surveyed but because fever nursing has been strangely sidelined. This book helps to retrieve fever nursing, nurses and their patients from the shadowlands of history and relocate it at the heart of health care history and contemporary debates in nursing. Dr Currie has done us a great service by reminding us of the relevance of fever nursing to contemporary debate in nursing; the essentials of care and the re-emergence of infectious diseases. I applaud Dr Currie's efforts and commend her book to you.

Professor Anne Marie Rafferty
Dean and Chair in Nursing Policy,
Florence Nightingale School of Nursing and Midwifery,
King's College, London
2004

# Preface

This book had its origins in a small local study of hospitals and nursing care in south Bedfordshire, written primarily for the benefit of pupil and student nurses I was teaching at the Luton and Dunstable Hospital, but also for local historians. There were no other texts on this subject. Of the twelve main institutions discussed, two were isolation hospitals and one was for smallpox patients. While carrying out this research in the early 1980s, I interviewed some doctors and former patients and a few nurses who had worked in isolation hospitals. Their testimonies, combined with primary source evidence, built up an interesting yet at times disturbing picture, so I was keen to pursue it further, at national level.

In the late 1980s, nurse education was due to be transferred into higher education and nurse teachers, like myself, were expected to become graduates. As I had not previously had the opportunity, I took a degree in English and Historical Studies at the University of Hertfordshire, and was then encouraged by the University of Luton, where I was a senior lecturer, to undertake a doctoral study. It was originally to include fever hospitals and fever nursing, and I duly collected information at record offices and libraries. Conference papers were given at Nottingham, Cambridge, Edinburgh, London and in Winnipeg. Through debate with delegates, and discussion with nursing, midwifery, psychology and sociology students I taught at diploma, degree and master's level, my own knowledge was enhanced. Unfortunately, for various academic reasons, fever hospitals and fever nursing could not form part of my thesis, so I determined to write this book.

Much of my career has been in nurse education, in clinical patient care and in the classroom, but my early career, as a registered general nurse (RGN), took me into private nursing, industrial work, theatres and accident service. The job which made the greatest impression on me was as the sister in charge of a special clinic for patients with what are now termed 'sexually transmitted diseases'. The stigma attached to those with, or suspected of having, these diseases was plain to see. Patients ranged from infants to elderly people; all needed care and understanding, a non-judgemental attitude, and a readiness to listen to their perspective in confidence.

Nursing has, therefore, given me the context for this book, which required considerable extra research. I hope that this study will become a source of reference for others seeking knowledge about the past, for without this we cannot progress.

Margaret R Currie
Leagrave, Luton
October 2004

## Note to the reader

Notes and brief references are appended to each chapter; full references appear in the Bibliography at the back of the book.

# Acknowledgements

When a doctoral thesis was first contemplated, in 1992, Dr Anne Marie Rafferty, then at the University of Nottingham, suggested the subject of fever hospitals and fever nursing, as it had not previously been researched nationally. Both Dr Rafferty and Dr Anne Hardy at the then Wellcome Institute for the History of Medicine, London, gave sound guidance in the initial stages. Although the direction of the thesis changed, they had set me on the right road which eventually materialised in this book. Dr Rafferty also read Chapters 4 and 5, and subsequently the whole book in draft form, as she had kindly agreed to write the foreword. My thanks are given to these two ladies for their academic advice and support.

I am grateful to the RCN Publishing Company Ltd, for allowing me to use information from four articles I published on fever and smallpox nursing in the *International History of Nursing Journal* between 1997 and 2001. The Editor of the *Dictionary of National Biography* (Oxford: Oxford University Press, 2004) has kindly permitted me to use some of the data from my article about Susan Villiers in this book.

Librarians and archivists at various libraries, record offices, museums and other institutions have been very helpful, especially Susan McGann, the Royal College of Nursing (RCN) Archivist, who placed relevant material at my disposal in Edinburgh, and reviewed Chapter 7. Dr Gerard Fealy, University College, Dublin, carried out research for me at An Bord Altranais (the Nursing Board) in Dublin, made relevant comments on Chapters 2 and 3 and also enhanced my general knowledge about Irish matters. Jonathan Evans, Archivist at the Royal London Hospital, gave me valuable advice about Edith Cavell and reviewed Chapter 6 about her, and Dr James Gray, retired Consultant in Communicable Diseases at the Edinburgh City Hospital, drew useful data to my attention. I have cause to thank all these people for their interest and authoritative guidance.

A number of other professional colleagues, in the United Kingdom and abroad, have shared their knowledge, and I owe them a debt of gratitude: Dr Elizabeth Adey, Lal Aubeeluck, Kevin Brown, Dr Catherine Burns, Sue Fox, Janet Graham, Dr Christine Hallett, Elizabeth Jenner, David Johnson, Dr Stephanie Kirby, Sandra Leggetter, Dr Brigid Lusk, Professor Joan xii *Acknowledgements*

Lynaugh, Dr Barbara Mortimer, Dr Rohinton Mulla, Dr Malcom Nicolson, Edith Parker, Lynda Taylor, Dr Pamela Wood and Sheila Zerr. Although I cannot mention everyone by name, I would like to thank, most sincerely, Olive Dodd (née Cowley), the first fever nurse I interviewed, who opened my eyes, and Harriet Cassells (née Thompson) who, trustingly, put her personal life and professional details about fever nursing in Belfast in my hands. I am indebted to them and to the other former fever nurses whose experiences have greatly contributed to the body of knowledge about fever nursing. Thanks are also due to them and, in some cases, their relatives for donating significant archival material to me, which will be transferred to the RCN Archives.

However, I owe the greatest debt to my husband, John Currie, not only for his unfailing support during the long gestation period of this book, but also for his ability to discuss issues and for his word-processing skills, without whose expertise this book would not have reached publication. Finally, the staff at Routledge, especially my Editor, Karen Bowler, and her assistant, Claire Gauler, have been unfailingly polite, pleasant and positive – I thank them.

# Abbreviations and common terms

| | |
|---|---|
| AIDS | Acquired Immune Deficiency Syndrome |
| BCN | British College of Nurses |
| *BJN* | *British Journal of Nursing* |
| BLARS | Bedfordshire and Luton Archives and Records Service |
| BNA | British Nurses' Association |
| BTTA | British Tuberculosis and Thoracic Association |
| CCSRN | Central Committee for the State Registration of Nurses |
| DMTSN | Dublin Metropolitan Technical School for Nurses |
| FNA | Fever Nurses' Association |
| FRCN | Fellow of the Royal College of Nursing |
| GNC | General Nursing Council |
| GP | general practitioner |
| HAI | hospital acquired infection |
| HIV | Human Immunodeficiency Virus |
| ICD | infection control doctor |
| ICN | infection control nurse/International Council of Nurses |
| ICNA | Infection Control Nurses' Association |
| IHMA | Infectious Hospitals Matrons' Association |
| IHMNA | Infectious Hospitals Matrons' and Nurses' Association |
| JNMCNI | Joint Nursing and Midwives Council for Northern Ireland |
| KCLA | King's College London Archives |
| LCC | London County Council |
| LFH | London Fever Hospital |
| LGB | Local Government Board |
| LMA | London Metropolitan Archives |
| MOH | Medical Officer of Health |
| M&B | May and Baker |
| MRC | Medical Research Council |
| MRSA | Methicillin Resistant Staphylococcus Aureus |
| NA | National Archives |
| NHS | National Health Service |
| NLI | National Library of Ireland, Dublin |
| PHS | Public Health Service |

| PRO | Public Record Office |
| PSA | Port Sanitary Authority |
| PTS | preliminary training school |
| RBNA | Royal British Nurses' Association |
| RCN | Royal College of Nursing |
| RCNA | Royal College of Nursing Archives |
| RFHA | Royal Free Hospital Archive |
| RFN | registered fever nurse |
| RGN | registered general nurse |
| RIDN | registered infectious diseases nurse |
| RLHA | Royal London Hospital Archives |
| RMPA | Royal Medico-Psychological Association |
| RSCN | registered sick children's nurse |
| SCM | state certified midwife |
| SRN | state registered nurse |
| SRO | Scottish Record Office |
| STD | sexually transmitted disease |
| TAF | toxoid antitoxin floccules |
| TB | tubercle bacillus (tuberculosis) |
| TUC | Trades Union Congress |
| VAD | Voluntary Aid Detachment |
| VD | venereal disease |
| WHO | World Health Organization |

## Common terms

**Endemic** – a disease commonly present in a localised area.

**Epidemic** – a widespread outbreak of a disease affecting many people simultaneously in a community.

**Pandemic** – a disease affecting people over a wide geographical area.

# 1 Introduction

> The zymotic [infectious] diseases replace each other; and when one is rooted out is apt to be replaced by others which can ravage the human race indifferently wherever the conditions of healthy life are wanting. They have this property in common with weeds and other forms of life; as one species recedes, another advances. By improving the hygienic conditions in which men live, you fortify them against infection; and further, by isolating the infected, the chances of attack are diminished.
>
> William Farr (1872)[1]

The warlike metaphors in the above quotation epitomise and emphasise the fear which accompanied epidemics of infectious disease in nineteenth-century Britain. The increasing importance of a sanitary environment to individuals, and isolation measures to protect Victorian society, were fundamental to the nation's health and efficiency. Those most intimately involved with the isolation of patients in hospitals were fever nurses. Fever nursing now seems a particularly quaint term, its one-time importance almost forgotten, its history inextricably bound together with fever hospitals; both evolved slowly over two centuries and yet, by the 1970s, both had virtually disappeared.[2] However, this study continues beyond then, due to international concern about bioterrorism in relation to the possible wilful dissemination of the smallpox virus. It is necessary to include this issue, and how British society is coping with the challenges posed by different forms of fever, such as new viruses, drug-resistant organisms and new strains of old infectious diseases because, as William Farr observed in 1872, 'as one species recedes, another advances'.[3]

General nursing and most specialist branches of nursing have been well documented, but fever nursing has, for some reason, been avoided; this book, therefore, essays to fill the gap. Two methodological tools were used in this book. Historical research was carried out using mainly primary sources, and empirical studies were undertaken using a descriptive case study approach. These methods enabled the collection of quantitative and qualitative data and helped to determine both the final content and the form in which the research was presented. They enabled the drawing together of apparently disparate elements into a cohesive study. It draws on archival sources, the work of contemporary scholars, medical, nurse and social historians, journals, books, newspapers, doctoral theses and web pages. Local examples are included, as they illustrate how central government measures were applied to local situations. The book mainly covers the nineteenth and twentieth centuries, except Chapter 4, which is specific to the period 1921–71. Chapter 5 begins in the eighteenth century, earlier than other chapters, while Chapter 8 continues into the twenty-first century. The establishment of fever hospitals and the development of fever nursing in Britain includes the whole of Ireland, despite partition in 1922. Although independence was gained by Southern Ireland then, it was still thought relevant to include what is now known as the Irish Republic. What happened in fever nursing in Ireland is important to understanding the development and decline of the specialism. The Introduction now continues with the concept and effects of fever, the locus of care and the development of the fever nurse's role.

## The concept and effects of fever

The word 'fever' derives from the Latin *febris*; its etymology is obscure and it was not in use until *c.* AD 1000. As late as 1933, the *Oxford English Dictionary*, defined it as 'A morbid condition of the system, characterised by undue elevation of the temperature, and excessive change and destruction of the tissues'. It also noted that it was a generic term for a group of diseases with the above characteristics, each of which have distinctive names: 'intermittent, puerperal, scarlet, typhoid, yellow, etc'. Although fever hospital/nest/patient/ward are mentioned, the term 'fever nurse' does not appear. Nevertheless, it is reasonable to assume that those who cared for patients with fevers became known as fever nurses.

Fever is then, associated with heat, hence the Latin *ferveo*, I burn, and from Greek origins, *pyrexia*, also meaning fever. Both are broad general terms, until associated with a particular infectious disease; in many cases, the fever is only secondary to the diseased state of the body. Fevers have existed since classical times. Wherever, and whenever, they occurred, the community was affected personally, but also nationally, because catastrophic epidemics reduced population levels. Thomas Malthus (1766–1834), in his *Essay on the Principle of Population* (1798), deduced that the Black Death, or 'Great Pestilence' (plague) in 1348–49, resulted in a loss of 30–45 per cent of the population. He regarded 'excesses of all kinds, the whole of train of common diseases and epidemics, wars, plague, and famine' as 'positive checks' on population.[4]

Factors known to have increased the incidence of infectious diseases were the immigration of people to Britain, the movement of the population within the country and urbanisation, which did not occur in Ireland. In the census of

1851, it was found that more people lived in towns than in rural areas in England and Wales. The living conditions of the poor in Britain were, at that time, often appalling. Inadequate sanitation and overcrowded houses exacerbated the spread of infectious diseases such as cholera, typhoid, relapsing fever, typhus and smallpox, but they were not confined to the poor: they could affect anyone. By 1860, Florence Nightingale had recognised that epidemics in children originated in schools.[5] Compulsory elementary education for children aged 5–10 years, introduced in England and Wales in 1880, intensified the problem, so that measles, scarlet fever, diphtheria and other conditions, such as ringworm, became even more widespread. Although most infectious diseases could be fatal and premature death was common, the classical infectious diseases, which mostly affected younger age groups, waned to such an extent over the twentieth century that, by 1988, they accounted for only 1 per cent of all deaths in Britain and in all developed societies.[6] It had taken many years, however, to reach this stage, due to ignorance.

Theories of infection causation differed before the late-nineteenth-century bacteriological advances. Various terms were used and meanings shifted. In medieval times, doctors adopted the Hebrew ritual of making lepers outcasts; it then became customary for certain groups of patients, such as those with rashes, to be isolated.[7] Because the causation of infection was so poorly understood, it was attributed to a number of causes. For instance, in 1641, the causes of pestilence were declared as:

1    Sin, which ought to be repented of
2    an infected and corrupted air, which should be avoided
3    an evil diet, which should be amended
4    evill humours heaped together in the body, being apt to putrifie, and beget a Fever, which must be taken away by convenient medicines.[8]

Due to the connotation of 'sin', infectious diseases were often regarded as divine retribution. Consequently, those affected were looked at askance, distanced and often stigmatised. Miasmas, the noxious vapours from organic matter, particularly human and animal waste, the wrong diet and the Galenic humours were also considered possible causes. Galen (AD 129–*c*.216) deduced that fever could result from an excess of yellow bile, black bile, phlegm or blood. Instead of the earlier Hippocratic treatment of fevers by starvation (feed a cold and starve a fever), Galen advocated energetic blood letting by venesection, to remove such excesses and restore humoral balance, not only when a fever was present, but also prophylactically.[9] In 1963, Michel Foucault, drawing on Herman Boerhaave's *Aphorisms* (1709), observed that the eighteenth-century concept of fever was not so much a sign of the disease, but resistance to it. Fever has, therefore, a salutary value, 'an excretory movement, purifactory in intention'.[10]

Infectious diseases were clearly different, but most continued to be known generically as fever diseases until the mid-nineteenth century; for instance, it was not until 1855 that diphtheria and scarlet fever were recognised as different conditions.[11] In the 1870s, some doctors were still using the term 'typhus' to describe all types of fever. To avoid confusion, the term 'enteric' was frequently employed from the mid-1870s, instead of typhoid, as it sounded so similar to typhus.[12]

Until the late nineteenth century, almost all epidemics were thought to arise through transmission from person to person, generated from, usually, filthy, local conditions. Notions of 'contagion' and 'miasma', of a more or less undefined kind, were combined with 'stench', commonly thought to be at the root of disease.[13] The bacteriological revolution is usually credited with changing medical thought and the dawn of a new modern age. For instance, in 1864, Louis Pasteur (1822–96) announced his germ theory of disease, which finally disproved the idea of disease causation through spontaneous generation, given the right circumstances. Robert Koch (1843–1910) demonstrated the existence of specific disease-causing organisms: anthrax in 1876, the tubercle bacillus in 1882 and cholera in 1883. A combination of careful observation and new scientific techniques advanced medicine. Observation of living patients at the bedside had resulted in diagnosis of some infectious diseases earlier, because they had particular identities and characteristics; those of diphtheria were published in 1826, typhoid in 1837 and typhus in 1849,[14] but they were not proved scientifically until later in the nineteenth century.

The pathological significance of heat in fevers may have been known since classical times, but little progress was made in calibrating body temperatures until the eighteenth century, when Gabriel Fahrenheit (1686–1736) developed an alcohol, then a mercury thermometer (1714), based on earlier models. His temperature scale ranged from a freezing point of 32° to 212°F boiling point. Despite the work of some continental scientists, there was little interest in the measurement of temperature until the mid-nineteenth century, when Carl Wunderlich (1815–77) published his manual of thermometry in 1868, *The Temperature in Diseases*, which was particularly useful in the differential diagnosis of fevers. Normal temperature (98.4°F) signified health and fluctuations indicated disease. Although the temperature had to be recorded at least twice daily, absolute accuracy was not essential: 'nurses and even relatives could take temperatures'.[15] However, as will be seen in Chapter 2, this was not necessarily wise in the mid-nineteenth century when nurses were drawn from the, often uneducated, servant class.[16]

## Locus of care

During the nineteenth century, the term 'fever hospital' gradually evolved into 'isolation hospital', and in some cases a 'hospital for infectious diseases'. In this book, these terms are used synonymously. Such nomenclature highlighted the disease aspect and, because of its associated stigma, hindered isolation. It was for this reason that Dr Thorne Thorne, Medical

Officer to the Local Government Board (LGB), advocated in 1881 that hospital names referring to diseases should be avoided.[17] Despite this advice, a confusing variety of names continued to be used for such institutions; smallpox hospitals, however, seldom had alternative names. As will be seen in Chapter 2, early fever hospitals were often hastily constructed temporary buildings, before necessity and legislation resulted in more permanent structures, particularly when workhouse fever wards could not cope in epidemics. Smallpox was different. The origins of institutions, specifically for this one disease, and the care that patients received is discussed in Chapter 5.

Hospitals in Britain were founded for different reasons. In some ways, the charitably endowed voluntary hospitals provided a model for municipal isolation hospitals, for example, in the medicalisation of care and the development of specialist roles for doctors and nurses. Before the Anatomy Act, 1832, acquisition of medical knowledge through dissection was strictly limited,[18] but it could be gained from living bodies. This was one of the reasons many voluntary hospitals were established in the eighteenth century, followed by specialist and children's hospitals, although their foundation also gave rein for the charitable impulse.[19] In the eighteenth century, the submission of a body could be regarded as 'docile' if it was committed to a medical institution, in much the same way as to a military, educational or industrial establishment. It might then be 'subjected, used, transformed and improved'.[20] Thus, docility came to be regarded as a prerequisite of patients, who were expected to accept meekly whatever care was available.

Access to patients' bodies improved knowledge and gave doctors the opportunity to take paying pupils, who duly deferred to them. Through working in an honorary capacity with the 'deserving poor' in voluntary hospitals, they met 'the great and the good', people in high society and the upper-middle classes, who had often founded them and still contributed to their maintenance, often by taking out subscriptions. When they or their families were ill, they would be cared for in their own home, but would consult these new experts. Consultants were, then, self-employed men with private patients, who 'walked the wards' of general hospitals in an honorary capacity, the élite of their profession. Small districts had different needs.

The cottage hospital movement began in England when the first one was established in 1859 in Cranleigh, near Guildford, Surrey, by Mr Albert Napper, a local medical practitioner.[21] General practitioners (GPs) in the new cottage hospitals began to carry out a similar role to consultants, particularly in surgery; long-stay medical patients were generally discouraged. Cottage hospitals provided a locus of care for respectable people of the artisan class, who did not have to travel to distant voluntary hospitals, nor did they have to enter the infirmary at their local union workhouse. Due to the risk of wound infections in the pre-antibiotic era and the possible spread of infectious disease, some groups of patients were excluded. For example, at Luton Cottage Hospital, which opened in 1872 with just three beds, the rules stated that patients suffering from pulmonary consumption, unless deemed urgent by the Medical Officer, were ineligible, as were 'cases of Mania, Epilepsy, Infectious and Incurable diseases'.[22]

Isolation hospitals were very different in that they were founded by local authorities, initially for the poor, in much the same way as workhouses. Patients, particularly children, rarely entered them willingly, and the doctors who provided medical care were paid employees of the local authority and often, therefore, regarded as inferior by self-employed doctors. Small hospitals managed with a non-resident local Medical Officer of Health (MOH), or sometimes a GP. Large hospitals, however, had their own resident medical superintendents, who were, in effect, consultants by virtue of their experience and specialist training; consequently, medical students were frequently sent there for clinical experience and ward rounds. Nevertheless, by 1907, one eminent doctor, at the University of Manchester, felt that 'in the minds of many ... there exists a strong prejudice against the fever hospitals'.[23]

It was in this context that the specialism of fever nursing developed through the nineteenth and twentieth centuries. It has become apparent during this research, that doctors in the nineteenth century were relatively helpless in the evolution of disease patterns. They 'affected epidemics no more profoundly than did priests during earlier times. Epidemics came and went, imprecated by both but touched by neither'.[24] Although the use of vaccines was significant, medical management was limited, hence fever nurses, who were trained to assist the doctor and obey orders, gradually played a more and more important therapeutic role in the patient's recovery.

## Development of the fever nurse's role

Florence Nightingale believed that observation of the sick by nurses was essential, but deplored the fact that it was 'little exercised'.[25] Gradually, technical innovations were introduced to provide objective, accurate results. Taking and recording the patient's temperature, using the Fahrenheit scale (32–212°F), was initially the doctor's role, but as the doctor was not constantly present, nurses assumed the task. Great emphasis was placed on this aspect of their work in lectures and at the bedside. Textbooks for fever nurses often carried pages of illustrations of temperature charts indicative of different febrile diseases, which reinforced their importance in diagnosis and prognosis. Excellent examples of temperature charts have been seen in patients' medical notes held in various record offices. It is clear that most nurses took a pride in this aspect of their work.

The glass thermometer, which contained mercury, was usually inserted under the tongue, but in young children it was placed in the axilla or groin and in infants, the rectum. Gradually, the term 'pyrexia' superseded the term 'fever', hence the still vague diagnosis of 'pyrexia of unknown origin', but children who have fits due to a raised temperature are still described as having febrile convulsions. The frequency of taking and recording the temperature was specified by the doctor in charge of the patient, but at least twice daily; the more pyrexial the patient, the more frequent the recordings. Such close attention took the nurse to the bedside, where any other changes could be observed, such as whether the patient was sweating and needed clean bedclothes, the changed character of a rash, obstructed respirations, or if the patient was no longer able to be roused. Means were taken to reduce temperature locally by free ventilation, reduction of bedclothes or use of a bed cradle. A free intake of water was encouraged and the bowels were kept open. Tepid sponging of the whole body was a frequent nursing measure. Hence, temperature control became part of the advances in clinical nursing.

The nurse in isolation hospitals may have assisted the doctor by monitoring the patient's condition and reporting any change, but essentially, the nurse's role was to provide basic nursing care, particularly while the patient was on bed rest, which could last for many weeks. This included feeding and the administration of fluids and prescribed drugs, hygiene, care of pressure areas, and any special measures relevant to patients with particular diseases. These could be relatively simple, like care of the mouth and eyes and application of poultices, or more complex, such as the application of lotions to prevent permanent disfigurement, particularly in smallpox, and ensuring that the airways of patients with tracheotomies, carried out as a result of laryngeal diphtheria, were kept open.

This discourse, concerning the concept and effects of fever, the locus of care and the development of the fever nurse's role, has been provided to further the reader's understanding of the following chapters, which trace the origins of the care of patients with infectious diseases in Britain from *c.*1800 to the early twenty-first century. Chapter 2 outlines the transition from community to hospital care, the consequent need for nurses and problems of retention which led to fever nurse training schemes. Chapter 3 focuses on state registration in relation to fever nursing, and on some issues in the inter-war years. A rationale is then given about the role of men in fever nursing. Health risks to fever nurses and a discussion on hospital admission versus care at home follow. A rare glimpse of care is provided in patients' perspectives. Pay and conditions of service are discussed before the effect of the National Health Service (NHS) is considered. Finally, the closure of fever registers is analysed before a conclusion is drawn.

Chapter 4 is devoted to first-hand narratives from former fever nurses in the period 1921–71, based on a study of fever nurse training carried out in 1994–95. Of the 130 self-selected sample of fever nurses targeted, 118 respondents returned the postal questionnaires, a 91 per cent response rate. Research continued until June 2002, as a further 9 respondents had a valuable contribution to make. Although social historians like Paul Thompson and Robert Perks advocate personal interviews to collect and record oral histories,[26] this method was not practical due to the scattered nature of the target population throughout the United Kingdom and the Irish Republic. However, the study gave the respondents an opportunity they welcomed to recall, analyse and reflect on their fever nurse training and nursing practice. The original study was published in 1998,[27] but this chapter draws on a more extensive range of data than was possible in a journal article.

Chapter 5 focuses on smallpox nursing, beginning in the eighteenth century, with the use of case studies. Chapter 6 is devoted to Edith Cavell, exploring her reasons for becoming a nurse, initially in fever nursing, and how this experience affected her subsequent career. Chapter 7 concerns two influential fever nurses, who made their mark on the specialism, in the twentieth century. Chapter 8 examines the consequences of closing the fever registers and most fever hospitals in the light of the single qualified nurse. Consideration is then given to the wisdom of isolation hospitals. Infection control nursing is then reviewed in the context of changing disease patterns and possible bioterrorism; it brings the book up-to-date. Chapter 9 draws the book to a conclusion.

## Notes and references*

1 W. Farr, Compiler of Abstracts (1839–79) at the General Register Office, London, in his annual letter to the Registrar General in the Thirty-Fifth Annual Report of the Registrar General of Births, Deaths and Marriages in England (abstract of 1872), 1874, C 1155, p. 224.

2 Regional centres remain, but their work, often involving infectious diseases imported from abroad, receives little publicity.

3 Farr, op. cit.

4 Anderson (1996), pp. 29, 256. Malthus' 'preventive checks' on population included celibacy or delayed marriage.

5 Nightingale (1969[1860]), p. 139.

6 Halsey (1988), p. 399.

7 Baly (1980), p. 20. See also Risse (1999), pp. 173–79, in which the author explores 'views of leprosy and the construction of stigma'.

8 Sherwood (1641), p. i.

9 Porter (1997), p. 75. Galen's theories held sway into the early nineteenth century.

10 Foucault (2003 [1963]), pp. 219–20.

11 Pelling (1978), p. 98.

12 Hardy (1993), p. 153.

13 Ranger and Slack (1992), p. 3.

14 Hardy (2001), pp. 5, 25.

15 Porter (1997), pp. 344–45.

16 Dingwall, Rafferty and Webster (1988). Chapter 1, 'Nurses and Servants', provides a background for this topic.

17 LGB (1882) Tenth Annual Report of the Local Government Board 1880–81, *C3290 Use and Influence of Hospitals for Infectious Diseases*, London: HMSO. (The Medical Officer's name is correctly cited as Dr Thorne Thorne.)

18 Richardson (1989).

19 Prochaska (1988).

*———
Full references appear in the Bibliography.

20 Foucault (1991[1975]), pp. 136, 314.

21 Emrys-Roberts (1991), p. 4.

22 Currie (1982), pp. 50–52.

23 A. K. Gordon (1907) 'The Position of the Isolation Hospital in the Training of a Nurse', *British Journal of Nursing*, 26 January: 65.

24 Illich (1990[1976]), p. 23.

25 Nightingale (1969[1860]), p. 105.

26 Thompson (1988); Perks (1992).

27 M. R. Currie (1997–8) 'Fever Nurses' Perceptions of their Fever Nurse Training, 1927–71', *International History of Nursing Journal*, 3(2): 5–19. The data include some audio tapes and one video recording.

# 2 Institutions and the evolution of nursing care

> Nursing is largely a woman's occupation and the women who nurse for gain are part of the female labour force in the community. They have an economic as well as a professional and humanitarian role. Many are also wives and mothers whose gainful employment has social implications.
>
> Charlotte Searle (1965)[1]

## Introduction

In early-nineteenth-century Britain, fever hospitals were the only institutions founded, through the Poor Laws, specifically for the physically ill. They were not primarily for their patients' benefit; the aim was isolation of the sick, rather than the provision of care. The main workload was borne by women; fever nursing, therefore, arose as a specialism out of necessity to ensure the needs of patients were met. The accommodation for those affected by infectious diseases was determined by a number of factors, including the size of the local population, the available resources, legislation and demographic change. Undoubtedly, fear and panic, generated by the virulence of a particular fever and its rapid spread in the local community, was usually the main factor which spurred the local authority to establish some form of fever hospital, or fever ward, often in the local workhouse.

In 1961, Erving Goffman described prisons and asylums as 'total institutions'; inmates were removed from a 'home world', stripped of their identity and possessions and, in many institutions, deprived of the privilege of having visitors.[2] Patients in isolation hospitals were often in a similar situation, with their nurses, technically, their guardians as much as providers of care. Before these hospitals were established, and even when they were, most people, particularly children, preferred to be nursed at home, however humble the conditions.

## Nursing care in the community

Traditionally, knowledge about fevers, rashes and remedies was handed down by word of mouth from generation to generation, now termed 'received wisdom'. Reciprocity of care, neighbours helping each other in adversity, was equally important. From the late eighteenth century, industrialisation and urbanisation in England and Wales, and in Scotland, meant that these benefits were often lost as people moved away from their rural roots. In Ireland, fever, famine and emigration, mainly to North America, had virtually the same effect. Ignorance could mean that the early signs and symptoms of fever (raised temperature and general malaise) were not recognised and, apart from smallpox, one rash was hard to distinguish from another. The problem was compounded by failure to summon a doctor soon enough, often owing to poverty. The houses of the poor were often squalid, overcrowded, seldom equipped with the basic necessities to nurse the sick, and there was rarely enough money for medical attention. In any case, doctors in private practice tended to work in more affluent urban areas in order to earn their living, so access to them was often difficult. Although sanitary reform began to improve living conditions and reduce the incidence of cholera and typhoid, it failed to address the spread of other infectious diseases. Diarrhoeal diseases were common in infants, leading to high infant mortality rates. Where there were horses and cattle, flies were attracted, now known to spread infection.[3]

Local MOHs were appointed in urban and rural areas to advise their local authority of epidemics of infectious diseases, problems with sanitation, or any other adverse influences on the health of the community. Some large urban areas found it necessary to appoint them in the early nineteenth century, under local powers, as was the case in Liverpool and the City of London; other large towns had appointed qualified medical men under the Public Health Act, 1848.[4] In London, 48 MOHs were appointed in 1856 as a result of the Metropolis Local Management Act, 1855, and others were appointed in all urban and rural sanitary districts in England and Wales under the Public Health Act, 1872.[5] However, the prevention and spread of infectious disease was really dependent upon the early detection and reporting of the problem to the local MOH. Until legislation was enacted, this was unlikely to happen.

Statutory notification was first introduced in England and Wales in the Public Health Act, 1875, in which cholera was made notifiable. Any local authority in Britain could introduce this measure. For instance, compulsory notification for infectious diseases was introduced in Edinburgh in 1880.[6] The Infectious Diseases Notification Act, 1889, was mandatory in London and permissive elsewhere in England and Wales, and the Infectious Diseases Notification (Extension) Act, 1899, made notification compulsory throughout England and Wales (see Appendix 1). The benefit of these Acts was that the MOH was immediately informed about the presence of certain diseases in his district,[7] and could take necessary action. Venereal diseases, now termed sexually transmitted diseases (STDs), have never been listed in this legislation, although successive Contagious Diseases Acts, 1864, 1866, 1869, which required the compulsory medical examination of prostitutes in military towns and naval ports, served this purpose. Lock hospitals (from the medieval locques, meaning lepers) were used to detain women forcibly. Fear, mainly of syphilis, created alarm in the community, which, together with outrage at their forcible detention, resulted in controversy; campaigns were launched to revoke the Acts and they were finally repealed in 1886.[8]

During the second half of the nineteenth century, nurses began to be employed in the community to help the sick, such as parish nurses funded by local churches. Following Queen Victoria's Golden Jubilee in 1887, general nurses with extra training, including care of patients with infectious diseases, were appointed Queen's nurses in her honour.[9] Following Joseph Lister's battle against hospital sepsis and his use of carbolic acid (phenol) to prevent wound infection in the mid-1860s, nurses began to be taught the importance of hygiene in hospital and in the home. Queen's nurses strived hard to bring the new Listerian hospital standards of hygiene to households struggling, often through no fault of their own, against filthy conditions inside and around the home. Queen's probationers in Dublin had five questions on 'Fever' in their examinations in December 1892 and March 1893, which mentioned patients with smallpox, measles and scarlatina, and one question that asked 'How would you arrange a sick-room for the treatment of an infectious patient?' [10]

Horace Sworder, part-time MOH to the Borough of Luton, had seen the problems that infectious diseases, such as scarlet fever and diphtheria, wrought on families nursing the sick at home, often in unhygienic circumstances; in 1893 he published a simply worded, 82-page guide,[11] but it would also have been useful for nurses in the first isolation hospital established in the town that year.[12] The middle classes, who usually lived in more spacious surroundings, were likely to cope better with infectious disease; a doctor in private practice would be called, maids could act as nurses, or if a professional nurse visited, the maid could assist her. Whether the family was poor or 'well-to-do', there was a reluctance to surrender feverish relatives into isolation hospitals when they were established as, initially, most were intended for paupers and had a poor reputation. This could lead to concealment of infectious disease and less chance of recovery, although, even when a patient was admitted to hospital, there was always the risk of contracting another, perhaps, more serious disease.

## Demographic change

Various factors determined the prevalence, morbidity and mortality rates of infectious diseases, but the larger the community, the greater the impact of an epidemic and the greater the urgency to separate the infected from the healthy. The census of 1851 showed that, for the first time, more people in England and Wales lived in towns than in rural areas. A survey carried out in 1908 in the British Isles, published in 1909, revealed great disparities in population between the four countries (Table 2.1).

*Table 2.1* Population change in England, Wales, Scotland and Ireland, 1851 and 1908

| Year | England | Wales | Scotland | Ireland |
|------|---------|-------|----------|---------|
| 1851 | 16,926,348 | 1,001,261 | 2,888,742 | 6,552,385 |
| 1908 | 33,472,252 | 1,876,528 | 4,826,587 | 4,364,226 |

Source: *Public Health and Social Conditions: Statistical Memoranda and Charts prepared in the Local Government Board relating to Public Health and Social Conditions*, Cd 4671, London: HMSO, 1909.

It is clear that, while England had seen the greatest growth, the population of Ireland had diminished. In fact, in 1841 there was an even higher population of 8,198,124 persons.[13] The potential for epidemics may have been greater in England, particularly in London, due to the larger population, and because it was a major port, but other factors, such as overcrowding in slum dwellings have to be taken into account, a situation not peculiar to that city. Failure to address the problem of epidemics could threaten industrial, military and imperial might if too many lives were lost. Fever hospitals were established around heavily populated urban areas in nineteenth-century Britain, but were rarely speedily established in rural communities, due, mainly, to poor understanding of the causation and transmission of infection and financial constraints.

## Growth of isolation hospitals and development of nursing care

Founded in 1801, the Liverpool Fever Hospital was the first English hospital specifically for infectious diseases, other than smallpox. London was then the largest city in the world and expected to set an example to the nation and to the British Empire, yet it had only two specialist hospitals for infectious diseases: the 100-bed Smallpox Hospital in Highgate, founded in 1741, and the London Fever Hospital, with 182 beds, opened in 1802. These were voluntary institutions, mainly for paying patients, although contracts were later taken out by Poor Law Unions. Some early fever hospitals were euphemistically and optimistically referred to as 'houses of recovery', as in London, Manchester and Newcastle-upon-Tyne, which set up such institutions between 1802 and 1804. The austere stone three-storey House of Recovery in Newcastle, built outside the town walls in an 'airy and retired situation', survives.[14] Institutions were established according to local need. For example, the county town of Bedford had its own fever hospital in 1847,[15] while the, then, smaller market town of Luton managed with a fever ward, opened in 1850, at the 1836 union workhouse.[16]

The establishment of virtually all isolation (and smallpox) hospitals was dependent on local authority provision and, therefore, decidedly slow in comparison to voluntary hospitals, 250 of which had been founded by the

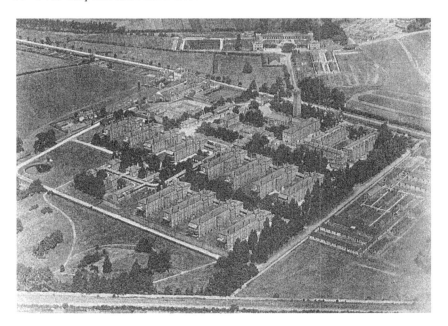

*Figure 2.1* Aerial view Brook Hospital, Woolwich, London County Council, 1935.
London Metropolitan Archives

middle decades of the nineteenth century. However, increased public health legislation gradually changed this balance.[17] In London, the Metropolitan Poor Act, 1867, empowered the Poor Law Board to combine parishes and to provide fever and smallpox hospitals and asylums for paupers. This Act led to the creation of the Metropolitan Asylums Board (MAB) as one hospital authority for the whole of London, superseded by the London County Council in 1930. The MAB set up nine acute fever hospitals and the temporary Fountain Fever Hospital, surrounding London in the period 1870–99, and it became the largest and most efficient such organisation in the world (Figure 2.1). The Latin motto *miseris succurrere disco* on the MAB Coat-of-Arms, 'I learn to succor [*sic*] the wretched',[18] was to become particularly apt for fever nurses.

In 1871, the Local Government Board took over from the Poor Law Board in England and Wales. The Poor Law (Amendment) Act, 1876, waived charges for non-pauper patients admitted to MAB fever hospitals. However, local authorities were reluctant to establish isolation hospitals and very few did so, as it was optional under Section 131 of the Public Health Act, 1875. Section 124 of the same Act referred to 'anyone with a dangerous infectious disorder without proper lodging or accommodation or on board a ship or vessel', who could be removed, with certain provisos, as long as there was a suitable place. In 1879, the LGB reported that 'means for isolation of some sort or other were possessed by 192 urban, 87 rural and 17 port sanitary authorities out of a total of 1,593 such authorities in England and Wales'.[19]

As will be seen in Chapter 5, in the late nineteenth century, the MAB in London made provision for the isolation and care of smallpox patients in three ships moored in the Thames' estuary. Other ports made similar provision for a range of infectious diseases within floating hospitals. Port Sanitary Authorities (PSAs) were introduced into Britain in 1872, as an alternative system to quarantine, to prevent infections being imported via the coast; it was known as the 'English system'. Quarantine was unpopular; it demanded a minimum of 40 days' isolation and exclusion, which was not only costly, but also against British liberal principles. Although a Quarantine Act was passed in 1800, it dealt mainly with the construction and maintenance of quarantine stations in major ports. The Quarantine Act, 1825, dealt specifically with vessels travelling from ports where the plague or yellow fever 'or other infectious disease or distemper highly dangerous to the health of His Majesty's subjects' was known to exist. The English system concerned infectious diseases not covered by the 1825 Act, including smallpox, typhoid, scarlet fever and measles. Ships which had visible signs of the disease on board, as determined by a medical inspector, were required to be disinfected and the sick removed to an isolation hospital. The crew and passengers who did not manifest any symptoms were required to be monitored after disembarkation. Quarantine was not abolished until 1896, hence the two systems coexisted for over 20 years.[20]

The River Tyne PSA (Jarrow Slake) was one of the few such bodies to provide 'efficient isolation accommodation in the actual waterway of the port over which their jurisdiction extends'. The hospital, which opened in 1882, was built on 10 cylindrical pontoons, 70 feet in length and 6 feet in diameter, with a floating power equal to 535 tons (Figure 2.2). It supported a strong iron framework with a deck of creosoted timber on which were created three main buildings, each consisting of one six-bedded ward and one four-bedded ward, divided by a nurses' room and bathroom. Each ward had a scullery and a water closet. A gangway ran round the sides and the ends of each building where it butted onto the river. A small mortuary, behind the central ward, 'appears perilously near the ward windows, the clear distance being only three feet'. A second floating hospital, which was attached by a gangway, previously used for cholera, was used for administrative purposes.[21] An internationally recognised yellow and black flag was flown when there was infection on board.

It is clear that this floating hospital was used for a range of infectious diseases during her existence from 1886 to 1930, when she was dismantled. For example, in 1902, the following infectious diseases were reported during the voyage, or on or after arriving in port: smallpox and suspected smallpox, measles, enteric fever (typhoid), scarlet fever, diarrhoeal diseases, malarial fever, dysentery and influenza. Of these, 17 cases were removed to this hospital. The other 51 cases admitted that year were patients with smallpox, from districts without any hospital provision, as the floating hospital had been reserved for that disease that year. Port officers boarded 2,323 vessels

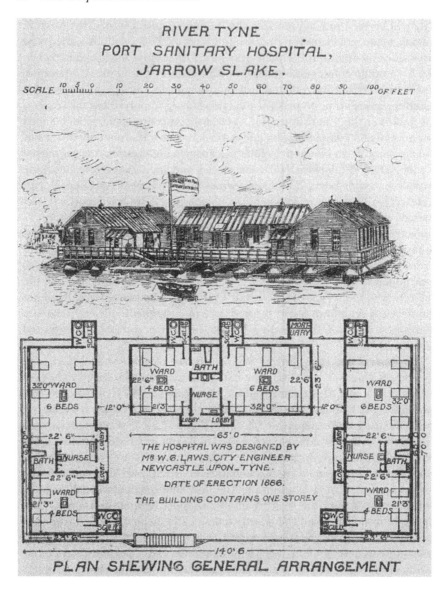

*Figure 2.2* River Tyne Port Sanitary Authority Hospital, Jarrow Slake, 1886.
British Library. Source: H.C. Burdett (1893), *Hospitals and Asylums of the World, Portfolio of Plans*, London, Scientific, p.80.

because they came directly, or indirectly, from infected or suspected ports; of these, 1,875 were directly or indirectly from infected ports. In 1902, the number of emigrants passing through the Tyne Port was 2,434, an increase of 412 compared with the previous year. All emigrant vessels were visited by the inspectors on arrival and then kept under supervision while in port. As in former years, information about emigrants 'debarking' [*sic*] and proceeding overland to other ports was forwarded to the MOHs of the respective ports. The River Tyne Port MOH had visited 46 vessels from infected or suspected ports due to sickness on board being reported or suspected. On 8 August 1902, a Lascar (a sailor from the East Indies) who had arrived in the port, died in Newcastle Royal Infirmary from suspected bubonic plague. Although the diagnosis was not confirmed from specimens sent to the LGB, all precautions were taken as if the case was actually one of plague, and 24 vessels were fumigated for the destruction of rats.[22]

It is evident that the potential for epidemics in Britain was minimised by the national systems in force, administered locally. Little is known about the nurses on board this floating hospital, although they would quickly have gained knowledge through practical experience. The architect clearly paid attention to the LGB directive to provide at least three separate wards for different diseases, and ensured that the nurses of each ward did not have to come into contact with other patients or nurses, thereby obviating or reducing the risk of cross-infection. The reason for the Lascar, who died from suspected bubonic plague, being nursed in Newcastle Royal Infirmary, may have been that he was admitted for some other reason and was in the incubation stage before the disease was suspected, or that the floating hospital was full due to the serious epidemic of smallpox in 1902. In many respects this PSA was a model authority, but not all sanitary authorities recognised their duty to provide the efficient hospital accommodation the LGB was trying to achieve in England and Wales.

In 1882, Dr Thorne Thorne's 'Report on the Use and Influence of Hospitals for Infectious Diseases' was published as a supplement to the Tenth Annual Report of the LGB. The inquiry that gave rise to the report had been commissioned by the LGB in 1880 for two reasons: first, to consider the proper planning and construction of infectious hospitals, and second, their possible role in the spread of disease in the vicinity. Of a sample of 70 infectious hospitals visited by Dr Thorne Thorne in 1880–81, in which 150 different sanitary authorities were concerned, only 19 were purpose built, 21 were partly or entirely constructed of wood or iron, seven were workhouse infirmaries or general hospital wards, while the remainder were old villas, semi-detached houses and cottages which had been adapted for the purpose; a cotton mill and a former brewery had also been used. His key recommendation was that purpose-built isolation and infectious accommodation should be built in advance to prevent epidemics, instead of reliance on temporary huts, often completed too late.[23]

To this end, between 1876 and 1924, the LGB regularly published model plans of isolation hospital ward blocks for the benefit of local authorities, who copied them extensively, the main reason being that they would then qualify for a loan from the Board.[24] In any case, the large-scale architectural designs favoured by the MAB, and other large cities in Britain, were not suitable for smaller hospitals. Although Section 131 of the Public Health Act, 1875, stated that two or more local authorities could combine to provide a common hospital, this seldom happened quickly. Section 132 of the same Act permitted local authorities to recover any costs incurred in a hospital or temporary place, 'deemed to be a debt', from patients, but not paupers, within six months of discharge, or 'in the event of his dying in such hospital or place'. The Isolation Hospitals Act, 1893, Section 3, empowered county councils to require local authorities to build isolation hospitals. It was this measure, combined with the Notification Acts, 1889, 1899, which led to a further growth in isolation hospitals. Many authorities, however, took advantage of the Public Health Act, 1875, Section 131, to provide 'temporary places' for the reception of the sick. These included ships, tents and wooden sheds, usually clad in corrugated iron; houses could also be commandeered in an emergency.

Nursing care had to be adapted according to circumstances, sometimes in very primitive conditions. For example, at Spittlesea, the Borough of Luton's isolation hospital, opened in 1893 on a remote hill-top site owned by the corporation (now occupied by Luton Airport), water was supplied by a water cart and the only available means of lighting was by oil lamps. Water and electricity were laid on only in 1906 (Figure 2.3).[25] Like Luton, most small local authorities made minimum provision initially and added buildings piecemeal over subsequent years. The LGB, however, set high standards; for instance, it insisted that new hospitals should enable the treatment of at least three diseases at once, the commonest, scarlet fever, usually being

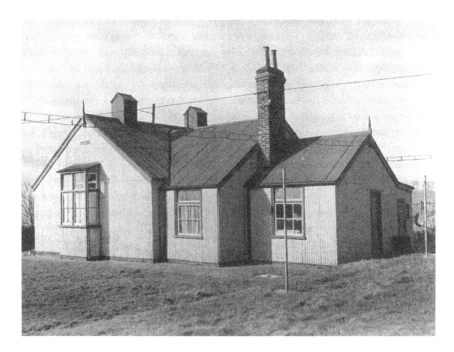

*Figure 2.3* Spittlesea Isolation Hospital, Luton, *c*.1906. *Luton News*

allocated more space. As typhoid fever and diphtheria required the most nursing care, the blocks contained a maximum of 12 beds. It was common practice for wards to be named after infectious diseases, although flexibility was essential as some epidemics produced more patients with a particular disease. Tents were often used to provide additional accommodation. Wards were initially built on a pavilion plan that extended out from either side of a duty room or rooms. Windows on both sides allowed cross-ventilation. Large hospitals had long parallel rows of wards, but small hospitals usually had a more friendly arrangement with the wards arranged around a central green or garden. Service buildings included a laundry and disinfector and, after the Infectious Diseases (Prevention) Act, 1890, a mortuary, because the bodies of those who had 'died from infectious diseases should be removed from the hospital directly to the place of burial'.[26]

As more was learned about the spread of infection and the course of infectious diseases, plans became more refined and better facilities were provided. Sanitary annexes were usually sited at the outer ends of wards, separated by ventilated lobbies, with hand-washing basins. Portable baths were in use in some hospitals, as it was thought better, at one time, for patients to be bathed next to their bed. However, it became more common for a special discharge block to be built, which enabled contaminated clothing to be removed by the patient in one room, proceed into the bathroom for a thorough disinfectant cleansing and then transfer into the outer room to don a complete set of clean clothes. In the early twentieth century, a new design was introduced – the cubicle isolation block. This was ideal where the patient's diagnosis was uncertain and where a greater degree of isolation was thought necessary,[27] particularly when other diseases became notifiable, such as plague (1900) and acute poliomyelitis and tuberculosis (1912) (see Appendix 1).

Pulmonary tuberculosis, commonly referred to as TB, from the causative organism, the tubercle bacillus, discovered by Robert Koch in 1882, was a common cause of mortality, particularly in young adults, although the incidence of the disease began to decline from 1870, despite increasing urbanisation. Between 1851 and 1910 almost 4 million deaths in England and Wales were registered as due to TB, 13 per cent of the total mortality rates. Although sanitary authorities had had the power to provide sanatoria, tuberculosis dispensaries, shelters, tents, medical assistance and other resources for persons believed to have TB, it was little used.[28]

There had been various attempts by diverse bodies to make some provision, but there was not a nation-wide chain of sanatoria. However, the National Insurance Act, 1911, included a 'sanatorium benefit' clause (Section 8 (I)(b)), which provided for treatment in sanatoria or other institutions for insured persons above 16 years, which, together with notification, meant that more tuberculous patients were likely to be admitted to fever hospitals. A sum of £1.5 million was provided through this Act to construct sanatoria.[29] Some local authorities designated specific wards for this purpose

*Table 2.2* Number and types of institutions, beds in each class and average
number of beds in England and Wales, 1914

| No. and type of institution | | No. of beds | Average no. of beds |
|---|---|---|---|
| 755 | Fever hospitals | 31,149 | 41 |
| 700 | Poor Law infirmaries | 94,001 | 134 |
| 594 | General hospitals | 31,329 | 53 |
| 363 | Smallpox hospitals | 7,972 | 22 |
| 222 | Special hospitals | 13,654 | 62 |

Source: *Forty-fourth Annual Report of the Local Government Board, 1914–1915, Part III – (a) Public Health and Local Administration*, London: HMSO, 1916, Cd 8197, pp. 26–27.

in their existing isolation hospital, or changed its use to include a purpose-built sanatorium, while others founded a new sanatorium on a different site. For example, Bedfordshire established its sanatorium at Mogerhanger in 1921, under the control of the county council, distant from isolation and smallpox hospitals managed by smaller local authorities in the county.

As the number of patients admitted with infectious diseases rose, the demand on beds and staff increased and fever nurses needed to learn about a greater range of problems. By 1914 fever hospitals were the largest single type of institution in England and Wales (Table 2.2).

It is clear that legislation regarding the establishment of fever and small-pox hospitals had been effective, but in so doing had increased staffing problems. Due to the other types of institutions, particularly Poor Law infirmaries, which had a far greater number of beds, there was competition to attract staff, both probationers and trained nurses. As some large city fever hospitals had 500–1,000 beds, the average of 41 beds cited indicates that small hospitals had an extremely low number, which did not augur well for efficiency or proper nursing care.

Brian Abel-Smith commented on the variable size and quality of these institutions in 1964. For example in 1911, Liverpool had a splendid fever hospital for nearly a thousand patients, but large areas of England and Wales still made do with a primitive cottage or shed. Such hospitals often stood empty for months at a time, thus were frequently unfit for use when needed, and it was difficult to obtain trained nurses at short notice. As a result, it was not unknown for a patient to be left to the caretaker's attention. At least one local authority was sued for its 'scandalous arrangements', including Tunbridge Wells in c.1906.[30]

In Ireland, a few fever hospitals had been established, such as those in Dublin and Cork, within the first three years of the nineteenth century following a severe epidemic of fever and dysentery in 1799–1801. In 1818, an 'Act to establish Fever Hospitals, and to make other Regulations for Relief of the suffering Poor and for preventing the Increase of Infectious Fevers in Ireland' led to the establishment of a nation-wide system of state-funded fever hospitals, either by building or leasing. Pauper patients, therefore, received indoor relief under the Poor Law system. By 1835 there were at least 64 such institutions, and in the decade 1841–51, there are known to have been 222 temporary institutions and 122 permanent fever hospitals.[31] In early-nineteenth-century Ireland, as in other countries, the lack of nurse training was apparent. In 1817, the Hardwicke Fever Hospital, Dublin, found it necessary to issue 18 points concerning basic nursing care as guidance to nurses. In 1835, Dr Denis Phelan referred to nurses as 'ignorant'. He felt that numerous, valuable lives were lost and contagious diseases extended if not created. Nurses then were opposed to washing patients or changing their linen – and they excluded fresh air.[32] The main efforts seem to have been directed towards establishing more and more institutions, but there was no driving force to improve the standard of nursing care.

It was found that the established fever hospitals in Ireland were mostly too small to cope with a major epidemic. The Great Famine was a disaster of major proportions, not only for the people, but also for the authorities, who tried hurriedly to fill the gaps in accommodation when epidemics of typhus, relapsing fever, dysentery and scurvy broke out between late 1846 and early 1847. The solution was found in temporary fever hospitals; although little more than sheds, they treated *c.* 580,000 patients between July 1847 and August 1850. The sheer weight of numbers was so great that even then most fever victims did not enter a hospital during the Great Famine. Even the 130 union workhouses which existed in Ireland in 1847 failed to cope with the flood of paupers, many of whom were suffering from different fevers. For example, in early March that year, the Fermoy Workhouse in County Cork, which normally accommodated 800 persons, was inundated with 1,800 paupers. As the town did not possess a fever hospital, the sick and the healthy were all mixed together. Consequently, of the 2,294 persons admitted since 1 January 1847 and not discharged, 543, or nearly 24 per cent, had died within two months.[33] The demand for women to care for these unfortunate people must have been very great, but it is likely that, even with the help of nursing nuns, only the most basic of nursing care was possible for the majority of those affected.

During the nineteenth century, a medical debate focused on the links between typhus, relapsing fever and food supplies. The debate is important in this context: it determined not only the type of care fever patients received in Ireland, but also where they were nursed. If, for example, typhus and relapsing fever were caused by hunger, it was not necessary to separate the sick from the healthy. The Dublin physician, Dr Dominic Corrigan, based his case on a detailed analysis of the famished over the previous centuries. By 1846 he had concluded that fever was caused by famine. Dr Henry Kennedy, physician at Cork Street Fever Hospital, Dublin, pointed out, however, that there had been many 'feverish years' when food had been plentiful. His view was supported by his colleague, Dr Robert Graves. Despite this logical conclusion, the Commissioners of Health in Ireland declared in 1852 that 'experience had shown that the scarcity of food in Ireland, if of any duration, had been inevitably followed by an epidemic of Fever'.[34] This understandable, but erroneous, belief resulted in a policy of nursing fever patients in general hospitals with those who were not infected, thus allowing the spread of disease.

It was a change in medical opinion at the end of the nineteenth century that led to the foundation of the Purdysburn Fever Hospital in Belfast in 1906. Doctors realised that, from a medical and scientific viewpoint, medical and surgical patients should not be cared for in the same building as fever patients, who were, in any case, reluctant to go into the Poor Law Union Workhouse (1841), where there was purpose-built fever accommodation. Belfast (like Dublin) had made use of makeshift accommodation earlier, including temporary sheds and rented houses, but it had been inadequate for the overwhelming numbers of patients needing attention in epidemics, even with the provision of Frederick Street Hospital in 1815.[35]

In Scotland, infectious diseases caused havoc in the cities. When the Royal Infirmary was opened in Glasgow in 1794, 'it became in effect the fever hospital for the city'. Due to frequent epidemics of typhus, smallpox and rarer invasions of cholera and relapsing fever, other measures had to be taken. Fever sheds were used from time to time and temporary district hospitals were hastily constructed in the suburbs. In 1847, typhus caused major problems. The city's old Town Hospital was converted to a fever hospital and fever sheds were provided in Anderston by Barony Parish. A total of 1,254 beds were provided and 11,425 cases were treated.[36] The emphasis was clearly on shutting away those infected, rather than on nursing care, which was unlikely to have been of a high standard due to poor conditions and the type of woman willing to volunteer. In 1865, when Kennedy Street Fever Hospital opened, the Superintendent, Dr J.B. Russell, wrote:

> At present nursing is the last resource [*sic*] of female adversity. Slatternly widows, runaway wives, women bankrupt of fame and fortune fall back on hospital nursing. When on a rare occasion a respectable young woman takes to it from choice, her friends most likely repudiate her and her relatives resort to various means of concealing her whereabouts.

Of 35 nurses engaged between 1865 and 30 April 1866, only 8 remained; the following reasons were given for the loss of 27 nurses:

| | |
|---|---|
| Dismissed for drink | 7 |
| Inefficiency | 5 |
| Dishonesty | 4 |
| Ill-using patients | 1 |
| Bad temper | 1 |
| Left of their own accord | 6 * |
| Died | 3 |

* Glad to be rid of some of them[37]

These data contribute to the growing evidence that fever nursing, like general nursing, needed to transform women from the servant class, often of ill-repute, into respectable professional nurses. The Belvidere Hospital was established in Glasgow in 1877. When it was still in a primitive condition in 1875, the Corporation appointed an untrained nurse, Amelia Sinclair, a 44-year-old widow, as Matron, as it had failed to find a satisfactory trained nurse. She is credited with transforming the role and status of the fever nurse in Glasgow. For example, she was responsible for securing a purpose-built nurses' home in 1877 with bedrooms, lavatories and bathrooms, which made a big difference to the type of young woman willing to become a fever nurse. When the permanent fever hospital, with 390 beds, was opened in 1887 at a cost of £76,167, Mrs Sinclair continued in post. Gradually, a more intelligent, better educated class of woman was attracted. Mrs Sinclair arranged for lectures to be given by the physician-superintendent and introduced certificates of proficiency. By the end of the nineteenth century, Belvidere Hospital had a nurse training school, and was considered the best fever hospital in the city until Ruchill Fever Hospital opened in 1900.[38]

Edinburgh also coped with the plague, smallpox, typhus, cholera and typhoid, sometimes in makeshift accommodation,[39] but there does not appear to have been in Scotland the same early rush to establish fever hospitals as was the case in Ireland. The population of Scotland was not large in relation to England and Wales in 1851 and 1908 (see Table 2.1), and it continued to increase very slowly. In 1921 it reached 4,882,288 persons.[40] By 1922–23, practically every small burgh or district had its own or a combination isolation hospital, and cities with larger populations had established isolation hospitals with a far greater number of beds, as seen in Table 2.3.

*Table 2.3* Number of beds in isolation hospitals in some Scottish cities in relation to population, 1921

| City/isolation hospital | No. of beds | Population |
|---|---|---|
| Glasgow Burgh | | 1,034,174 |
| Ruchill | 814 | |
| Belvidere | 625 | |
| Shieldhall | 128 | |
| Knightswood | 70 | |
| | Total: 1,637 | |
| Edinburgh Burgh | | 420,264 |
| City Hospital | 831 | |
| East Pilton | 100 | |
| | Total: 931 | |
| Dundee | | 168,315 |
| King's Cross Fever Hospital | 196 | |
| Aberdeen | | 158,963 |
| City Hospital | 214 | |

Source: Census of Scotland, 1921 and *Burdett's Hospitals and Charities, 1922–23*

It is clear that the larger the city, the greater the need for adequate provision of isolation hospital beds. These four large urban areas alone provided a total of 2,978 fever beds for a population of 1,781,716 persons; of these, 58 per cent lived in Glasgow.[41]

There can be little doubt that these and similar hospitals provided a source of employment for women who became nurses. Relatively little detailed evidence has been found about what form the nursing care took in early British fever institutions, although, as was seen in Glasgow in the 1860s, many of the women were unsuitable. Close parallels may be drawn with the problems that matrons of large voluntary hospitals experienced with unsatisfactory probationers in the 1860s to 1880s. After 1860, general hospitals began to train capable, privately educated middle-class women, some of whom were then willing to transfer their knowledge and skills as fever nurse leaders. The struggles they experienced in putting fever nursing on a professional footing may be attributed to the lack of elementary education which only became universal towards the end of the nineteenth century. Children were taught reading, writing and arithmetic, punctuality, obedience, respect for their betters - and to know their place, which made such a difference to the care in general and fever hospitals where hierarchies prevailed. Women from the servant class were now ready to accept very strict rules and regulations. Discipline had to be instilled to prevent cross-infection.

Under Dr Ker's medical superintendence (1903–36) and beyond, at the City Hospital, Edinburgh, at Colinton Mains, cross-infection was minimised by nurses attending patients with different diseases wearing pink or blue uniforms, according to the hospital area in which they were working (Figures

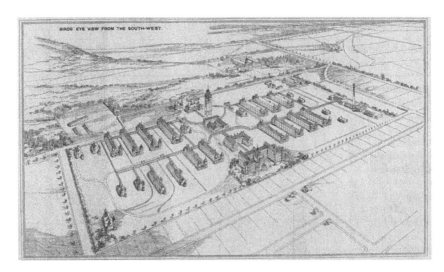

*Figure 2.4* Edinburgh City Hospital, sketch plan, 1896. Opened by King Edward VII, 13 May 1903. Temporary smallpox hospital beyond main hospital, left, and top right, Craiglockhart Poorhouse. Edinburgh City Libraries

2.4 and 2.5). Likewise, nurses on ambulance escort duties wore appropriately coloured uniforms according to the provisional diagnosis made by the general practitioner.[42] At the City Hospital for Infectious Diseases in Newcastle-upon-Tyne, in 1909, it was found necessary to issue a booklet with separate detailed rules, not only for every grade of staff, but also for patients and visitors. For example, the resident Medical Officer was obliged to give 'a

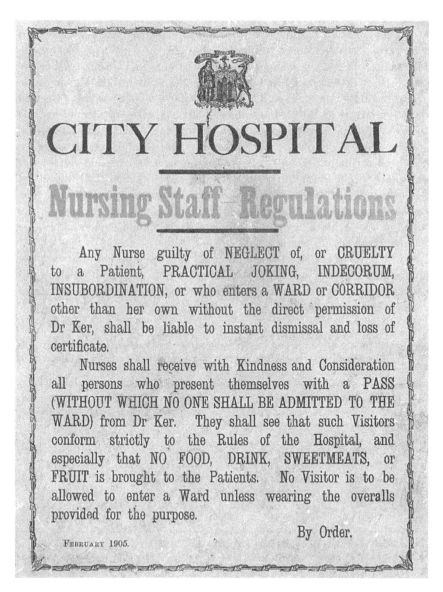

# CITY HOSPITAL

## Nursing Staff Regulations

Any Nurse guilty of NEGLECT of, or CRUELTY to a Patient, PRACTICAL JOKING, INDECORUM, INSUBORDINATION, or who enters a WARD or CORRIDOR other than her own without the direct permission of Dr Ker, shall be liable to instant dismissal and loss of certificate.

Nurses shall receive with Kindness and Consideration all persons who present themselves with a PASS (WITHOUT WHICH NO ONE SHALL BE ADMITTED TO THE WARD) from Dr Ker. They shall see that such Visitors conform strictly to the Rules of the Hospital, and especially that NO FOOD, DRINK, SWEETMEATS, or FRUIT is brought to the Patients. No Visitor is to be allowed to enter a Ward unless wearing the overalls provided for the purpose.

By Order.

FEBRUARY 1905.

*Figure 2.5* Edinburgh City Hospital Nursing Staff Regulations, 1905. This notice was permanently displayed in the wards. Edinburgh University Library

course of not less than twelve lectures to Nurses, with clinical instruction, between October and March', but he was not to permit nurses to administer hypodermic injections. The Matron was required to visit the wards 'at least once every twelve hours'. The longest list of 33 rules applied to the nurses who were to assist and control the probationers.[43]

## Staffing large and small hospitals

Setting up isolation hospitals had proved difficult, but staffing them, and more particularly, retaining staff, was even more of a problem. Before the Metropolitan Poor Act, 1867, was passed, Florence Nightingale had recommended that the proposed new MAB fever hospitals in London should be used for training nurses (as well as for medical instruction), as there were no trained nurses ready to assume the care of fever patients. Her advice was ignored and plans to establish the new institutions went ahead without this provision. Nursing nuns and assistant nurses, previously domestic servants, were used in the early epidemics.[44] The retention of assistant nurses was particularly problematic in the 1890s. Edith Cavell (1865–1915) was one of those who took up fever nursing then, only to leave after less than a year. The possible reasons for her becoming a fever nurse and the experience she gained at a large MAB hospital, which benefited her subsequent career, are examined fully in Chapter 6.

By 1882, the LGB was recommending one isolation hospital bed per thousand head of population.[45] Table 2.4 illustrates the extent to which this was achieved nationally and helps to explain the growing demand for fever nurses in the inter-war years.

*Table 2.4* Population, number of isolation hospitals, recommended and actual number of beds provided, and average number of beds per hospital in England and Wales, 1861–1968

| Year | Population (thousands) | Number of isolation hospitals* | Recommended no. of beds | Beds provided | Average no. of beds |
|------|------------------------|-------------------------------|-------------------------|---------------|---------------------|
| 1861 | 20,066 | 7 v         |        | 238    | 34 |
| 1891 | 29,003 | 5 v 353 p   | 29,003 | 10,757 | 30 |
| 1911 | 36,070 | 1 v 703 p   | 36,070 | 31,946 | 45 |
| 1921 | 37,887 | 1 v 888 p   | 37,887 | 41,593 | 47 |
| 1938 | 41,215 | 1 v 931 p   | 41,215 | 39,451 | 42 |
| 1949 | 43,785 | 315 NHS     | N/A    | 13,512 | 43 |
| 1968 | 48,511 | 25 NHS      | N/A    | 838    | 34 |

Sources: R. Pinker (1966) *English Hospital Statistics 1861–1938*, London: Heinemann; A. H. Halsey (ed.) (1972) *Trends in British Society since 1900: A Guide to the Changing Social Structure of Britain*, London: Macmillan; The Registrar-General's Statistical Review of England and Wales 1963 and Annual Abstract of Statistics 1991
v = voluntary, p = public
Notes: *Data for 1949 and 1968 show NHS hospitals; the recommended number of beds is no longer applicable

Table 2.4 shows that until 1921, there was a lag between the recommended number of beds and those provided. It also demonstrates that the number of isolation hospitals continued to grow in the inter-war years, when staffing all types of hospitals was difficult. As may be seen, by 1949 the number of isolation hospitals and beds had been drastically reduced. This was due to action by the new regional boards following the implementation in 1948 of the National Health Service Act, 1946. By 1968, the number of institutions and beds had been cut still further, but a few were retained. The number of institutions and beds had always dictated the number of staff required. One solution to recruitment and retention problems was to offer training; probationers, the cheapest form of labour, would then be under contract and less likely to leave.

## Fever nurse training

By the end of the nineteenth century, some hospitals in Britain were advertising lectures as an inducement to recruitment and a few of the larger institutions had already set up their own systems of fever nurse training, which varied from one hospital to another with regard to length, content, clinical experience available, and quality of teaching. As will be seen, Scotland began a national system of fever training from 1885. Edinburgh's second City Hospital, founded by the local authority, which opened in 1885, soon had a school for fever nurses. Certificates of proficiency and silver badges were awarded to successful candidates.[46] In 1899 it offered three years' training with lectures on physiology, hygiene, fever nursing, sick cooking and ambulance. Following satisfactory completion of the course and success in examination, a certificate was granted. This course was apparently oversubscribed; for example, in 1899, there were on average 150 applicants for the 30 vacancies. At the City of Glasgow Fever and Smallpox Hospitals, however, a Certificate of Proficiency in Fever Nursing was awarded after a two-year course of experience, lectures and a satisfactory pass in the written and *viva voce* examinations. In 1899, the wages of a probationer were £18–24 per annum, whereas in the same year at Edinburgh's City Hospital, the salary was £16 in the first year, £19 in the second and £22 in the third year.[47] Possibly, because there was more prestige attached to nursing in the capital city and greater demand for places, despite the longer course, a smaller salary was acceptable.

In 1981, Christopher Maggs, the nurse historian, cast more light on the development of nursing in Scotland through the Poor Law Service, including the specialism of fever nursing. His research showed that it originated in the Poor Law authorities (the Board of Supervision until 1885), thereafter the Local Government Board. The authorities were keen to rid the poorhouses of pauper nurses, untrained inmates, selected for nursing by the matron. 'All the pay they received [was] some beer and occasionally a half a crown [25p] a week'. In 1885 it was decided that part of the Medical Relief Grant for

Scotland could be used to encourage the employment of trained nurses in the poorhouses. As a result, an acceptable nurse–patient ratio was established, trained nursing was defined and the first state-sponsored register of sick nurses was set up in Scotland, 'thus anticipating the General Nursing Council by 35 years'. Under the 1885 regulations it was possible for fever and asylum nurses who had followed a two-year course to register as sick nurses, providing there was 'a medical presence' in the training hospital. Interpretation of the term 'training hospital' was left to the medical inspector, which led to non-general trained nurses on the register.[48]

Due to increasing recruitment problems in Scottish Poor Law hospitals, infirmaries and poorhouses, compounded by increasing competition for trained nurses by other institutions, changes were necessary. In 1907, training in general hospitals was lengthened from two to three years, including the time known in English hospitals as the 'trial period'. In 1911, the LGB scheme was extended to the 'other important area of Poor Law nursing provision, that of fever nursing'. A concession was made to fever nurse training, whereby probationers in that speciality could be taken on from 18 years of age, two years earlier than those in general nursing. At that stage, 20 infectious disease and fever hospitals under the jurisdiction of three county councils were then recognised by the Board. Maggs' data for the years 1907–14 includes four years (1907–11) not applicable to the new scheme of fever nurse training, yet in those seven years, of the 5,261 candidates for the final examinations, 2,135 were general nurses and 3,126 were fever nurses. Of these, 601 general and 1,006 fever nurses were granted LGB certificates as trained nurses.[49] The low pass rates testify to the high standards set by the Board, or perhaps, the poor education of the candidates.

In Ireland, the Fever Hospital and House of Recovery, Cork Street, Dublin, offered a two-year course in the closing years of the nineteenth century,[50] where Miss Carson Rae had been Lady Superintendent since 1896 (Figure 2.6). At this time, fever hospitals were benefiting from nurses who had had a comprehensive training. For instance, Miss Carson Rae had spent a year at the National Hospital for Paralysis in London and four years at the Westminster Hospital. She was also a qualified masseuse (physiotherapist), and worked for three years at St Marylebone Infirmary, initially as day sister-in-charge and afterwards as night superintendent.[51] Pupils were received for two years, during which time they had lectures in general medical and surgical practice, in addition to fevers. Some were given by Dr Day, the resident Medical Officer, clinical lecturer to the nurses. By 1895, Cork Street had already introduced an integrated scheme of nurse training whereby probationers in Dublin from these general hospitals: St Vincent's, Dr Steevens' and Jervis Street, and the Children's Hospital, Temple Street, were seconded 'for a course of three months in fever work'.[52]

The MAB in London was clearly determined to have high standards in the trained nurses it employed and in any courses it implemented. For instance, in 1894 it was decided that 'a nurse holding a certificate of 3 years' training

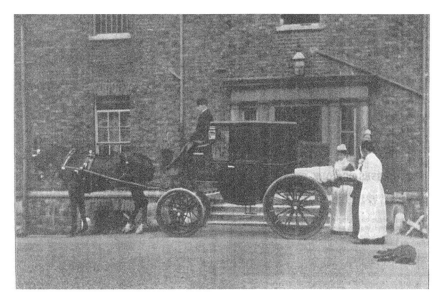

*Figure 2.6* The fever cab arriving with a fever-stricken patient at Cork Street
       Fever Hospital, Dublin, June 1895. British Library, Newspaper Library

at the London Fever Hospital is not qualified under the present regulations
to be appointed as a Charge Nurse in the Board's Fever Hospitals'.[53]
According to the London Fever Hospital records, the house directors resolved
on 24 September 1883, that 'nurses after 3 years service at the Hospital, may
be granted, if considered advisable, a certificate'. This was to be signed by
the chairman of the house directors and a physician.[54] Although the three-
year period may have included lectures as well as clinical experience, it was
clearly insufficient for the MAB in 1894.

Fever nurse training in MAB hospitals began only due to the high attrition
rate of first- and second-class assistant nurses. A return dated 7 November
1894 showed that in seven hospitals in the previous year, 158 nurses had left,
122 of whom had less than one year's service.[55] Despite improvements made in
conditions of service in 1892, there had been little change and in 1894, the
committee decided to recommend that the Board adopt a two-year experimental scheme of nurse training at the MAB Western Isolation Hospital.
According to Gwendoline Ayers, the MAB historian, nurse training in MAB
isolation hospitals was deferred until 1909, when a new 800-bed establishment
was opened at Carshalton. It was originally designed as a fever hospital, but
the need to provide for sick children in the London workhouses was greater,
and it opened as a children's infirmary.[56] There is evidence, however, that a
joint scheme of training was in existence in 1901, which may have started
earlier, between the MAB Western Isolation Hospital and Guy's Hospital.[57]

It is likely that the MAB, because of the possible implementation of a state
registration scheme, delayed instituting its own fever nurse training scheme.

However, at least one MAB fever hospital participated in another joint scheme of training in the early twentieth century. By 1904, an arrangement was in place for some probationers in Ireland, already undergoing general or children's nurse training, to be seconded for six months to the MAB North Western Hospital in Hampstead. They were employed as second-class assistant nurses, not probationers. They came in pairs from the same hospital; the first two, Marcella Sheridan (25) and Anna O'Donoghue (22), worked there from 29 April to 29 October 1904. They then returned to complete their general training at Jervis Street Hospital, Dublin. This arrangement continued until 6 June 1909, when it became more formal. Two nurses, aged 26 and 24 years, from the County and City Infirmary, Waterford, 'passed satisfactorily an examination in the nursing of Infectious Diseases', when they completed their time at the North Western. Records for the following year, in respect of two nurses, aged 25 and 27 years, from Jervis Street Hospital state, 'Certificate given for passing examination in Fever Nursing'. Other hospitals participated in this scheme, including the Children's Hospital, Temple Street, Dublin.[58]

The integration of fever nursing with general and children's nurse training was probably part of changes brought about in Ireland by the pioneering Dublin Metropolitan Technical School for Nurses, established in 1894. Participating hospitals, whose nurses attended lectures in anatomy, physiology, hygiene and invalid cookery, included the Hardwicke Fever Hospital. Nurses paid a one guinea fee (£1.05) and received a diploma when they passed the examinations; this was distinct from their hospital certificate. The Dublin Metropolitan Technical School Minute Book stated that the committee believed that 'the importance to the public of having a reliable standard of education for nurses cannot be overestimated, especially as to the management of infectious diseases and other matters relating to the public health'.[59]

As there were so many hospitals in Dublin, but relatively few fever hospitals by comparison, it was beneficial for Irish hospitals to collaborate with the North Western Hospital in London. The Irish nurses gained valuable clinical experience in infectious disease nursing, while the North Western gained extra 'pairs of hands'. At the end of the nineteenth century, Dublin, then the capital city of Ireland, had a larger population and was more important politically than Belfast. However, by 1901, the Union Infirmary, Belfast, had been functioning as a training school recognised by the LGB of Ireland for about three years; the wide curriculum included fever lectures and nursing.[60] Purdysburn Fever Hospital did not open until 1906. Between 1911 and 1933, provision increased from 168 to 575 beds.[61]

The Isolation Hospitals Act, 1893, Section 15, which did not apply to Scotland, Ireland or London, permitted a hospital committee, subject to any regulations made by the county council, to make arrangements for the training of nurses; two systems of fever nurse training then began to emerge, according to the size of the hospital. As there was then no national validating body to approve hospitals or courses for fever nurse training, there was little co-ordination or standardisation.

A seminal article published in the *British Journal of Nursing* (*BJN*), in January 1907, 'The Position of the Isolation Hospital in the Training of a Nurse', by Dr Alec Knyvett Gordon, a lecturer in infectious diseases at the University of Manchester, highlighted the fact that existing fever nurse training in a number of isolation hospitals left a lot to be desired. Many fever nurse candidates had to be rejected as they were undersized or anaemic (a fairly typical indicator of the health of the masses then). Gordon believed that probationers, not ward maids, should carry out 'menial' cleaning and that they should be well grounded in the principles of surgical cleanliness and aseptic technique for the safety of the patient. He showed his (probably justifiable) bias against what he termed the 'unsatisfactory type of fever hospitals', where generally the smaller the hospital, the more supervision the nurses needed, but the less they got. Although he acknowledged such institutions could offer excellent practice in ward work, this was not enough. In many instances, the nurses existed for the hospital, not the hospital for the nurses. Dr Gordon also observed that there was a 'strong prejudice against fever hospitals'.[62]

This article provoked Mrs Bedford Fenwick, the chief protagonist of state registration, into responding to many points in the next edition of the *BJN*, including the age that training could begin: 20–21 years in a fever hospital, but 23 years in a general hospital. She argued that if a girl could, under supervision, nurse scarlet fever and diphtheria, she was equally capable of attending patients with pneumonia and nephritis. Patients were far more frequently delirious in a fever hospital. She believed that the age limit appeared 'to be purely arbitrary, fixed by custom'. She also condemned the 'lack of discipline in a considerable number of fever hospitals'.[63] As a result of Gordon's and Fenwick's published comments, discussion was stimulated in the correspondence columns of the *BJN* concerning fever nurse training and the need for recognition of the status of the fever nurse. In June 1907, Mrs Fenwick pointed out that registration would become 'the sole mark of efficiency'.[64] Dr John Biernacki, Medical Superintendent of Plaistow Hospital, where a two-year fever nurse course for women with no previous experience, and a six-month course for nurses seconded during their general training, were already in existence, warned fever nurses that their salvation was in their own hands. He believed that their position was critical and urged them to unite to gain recognition under state registration.[65]

As a contributor pointed out in June 1907, general nurses, midwives, masseurs and others had their own associations, 'Why not fever nurses?'[66] Doctors were the first of the health professionals to achieve registration under the Medical Act, 1858, but not without a struggle. Midwives also had a battle to become recognised professional women, but eventually did so under the Midwives Act, 1902. Most fever nurses at that time, however, seemed to lack sufficient confidence to stand out alone for the cause of state registration. A number of medical superintendents (all male) appeared favourably disposed towards helping this particular female group to achieve its goals, perhaps because it was less liable to attract public censure than promoting the enfranchisement of women. It was in this climate of opinion and within the context of a series of campaigns to gain state registration, led by Mrs Fenwick, that the Fever Nurses' Association (FNA) was founded. Much of the primary source material for the following section is drawn from the *BJN*, as it became the unofficial organ of the new association.[67]

## The Fever Nurses' Association

The inaugural meeting was held on 10 January 1908. Dr Edward W. Goodall, Medical Superintendent of the MAB Eastern Hospital, was elected chairman of the provisional committee and Dr John Biernacki was elected as secretary. Dr Goodall moved 'That an Association be formed in the interests of Nurses in Fever Hospitals'. Dr Biernacki then gave a brief account of the movement, before Dr Brownlee, Medical Superintendent, City Hospital, Belvidere, Glasgow, gave a statement about the present conditions of fever nursing in Scotland. Although suggestions had been made to establish two associations, one of medical men and one of nurses, it was decided that there should be only one, 'since they were all working for a single object – the good of the nurses'. The title of the new body would be the Fever Nurses' Association. A provisional committee was formed with representative matrons and medical superintendents of some of the large fever hospitals and sanatoria in Britain, including the voluntary London Fever Hospital.[68]

The governing body, formed in June 1908, comprised 39 members: 20 medical men and 19 matrons and assistant matrons. Although most were from large British fever hospitals, three sanatoria were represented: Cardiff, Manchester and Salford. The MAB, which had a vested interest in a properly planned course for their own large hospitals, was particularly well served (see Appendix 2). The Articles of Association of the FNA showed that it intended to maintain a standard of training for fever nurses and keep a register of trained fever nurses. Some delegates brought with them experience of existing fever nurse courses set up in large hospitals under their own initiative. They were drawn from densely populated areas throughout Britain, among whom was Miss Carson Rae of Cork Street Fever Hospital, Dublin. This combination of medical men and senior female nurses was fairly unusual, but it provided the opportunity for such professionals to meet on equal terms and discuss policy issues. The interests of the MAB, the largest health authority in Britain, were ensured when Dr Goodall became the first president. Miss Susan Alice Villiers (1863–1945), a member of the first FNA Council, was able to use her nursing experience in positions of responsibility at different MAB fever hospitals for the benefit of the organisation.[69]

A scheme of training for isolation hospitals likely to be approved by the FNA was soon prepared. Provision was made for the training of nurses who were not general trained for a two-year course at a hospital with a minimum of eighty beds and at least one resident medical officer or visiting physician, who was a permanent officer in charge of the hospital. Probationers on this course should have at least eight lectures on elementary anatomy and physiology, four on medical and surgical nursing in relation to fever nursing and twelve on infectious diseases. For those already general trained, a one-year course was to be made available at a hospital with a minimum of a hundred beds and at least one resident medical officer. In this course, nurses should have at least twelve lectures on fever nursing and the common infectious diseases from a medical officer. In both cases, the hospitals were not to be solely for convalescents. The printed syllabus was to show the extent of the lectures, and the final examination was to be, as far as possible, in keeping with the syllabus. A schedule of ward instruction was to be provided in a case for the probationer to take with her to the wards, with items taught by the Sister initialled by her.[70] By 30 January 1909, the scheme had been submitted to the MAB for use in its isolation hospitals, but it was not approved until 31 July 1909.[71]

The FNA intended to encourage nurses who had completed two years' fever training to go on to general training, in order to become eligible in any future state scheme and obtain special recognition under state registration. It hoped to obtain recognition of fever training by general hospitals and believed that fever nursing should be part of general training. For fever nurses trained under their scheme, the FNA determined to shorten the general training by perhaps 6–12 months. Similarly, the fever training of general nurses trained at hospitals recognised by the FNA could be reduced from two years to one year. The FNA's decision to validate a two-year scheme was at odds with some Scottish hospitals, some of which, like the City Hospital, Edinburgh, had already implemented their own three-year course. It was to be the cause of much debate and ill-feeling later when the first General Nursing Councils (GNCs) were appointed.

The first annual general meeting, held on 24 May 1909, at the MAB offices, was attended by about eighty members, the majority being nurses. In his address, Dr Goodall, 'traced the origin of the modern fever hospital from the primitive "House of Recovery" . . . to the important position occupied by the fever hospital system . . . there were over 700 fever hospitals in the country, employing about 15,000 nurses'. Until the formation of the FNA, fever nurses had no organisation to voice their concerns or interests. For example, they could not take an effective part in the movement for state registration, neither could they lay claim to a 'reasonable measure of recognition under State Registration'. He explained that the FNA was in favour of the state registration of general trained nurses, but did not want to have those who were only fever trained registered by the state. The association felt that once a general trained nurse had obtained admission to the state register, she should be entitled to re-register her fever training as an additional qualification. For those who were only fever trained, the FNA provided a register and granted certificates. Trained fever nurses, who already had at least two years' experience in a fever hospital with a minimum of sixty beds, and general nurses who had six months' fever experience, were urged to apply for admission to the new Fever Register.[72] This plea in the *BJN*, through the auspices of Mrs Fenwick, is particularly significant. She had already set up a register for the British Nurses' Association (BNA) in 1887.[73]

In November 1910, Miss M. Drakard, Matron of Plaistow Hospital, West Ham, and a vice-president of the FNA, contributed an explanatory paper to the *Nursing Times* on the role of the nurse in fever hospitals. Readers of the *BJN* would already have been conversant with the proceedings of the FNA and the work undertaken by fever nurses. She pointed out that the first object of such hospitals was to prevent the spread of the various infections, not only 'among the people', but also within fever hospitals. The second object was the treatment and nursing of serious cases. She felt that fever hospitals, through their nurses, were doing great work not only for the state, but also in the saving of many lives that would previously have been lost. They also made it less likely that those who recovered would be free of conditions which could undermine their health. Prophetically, she observed that in small country hospitals, because of the nature of epidemics, the number of cases fluctuated in different seasons. This she felt was hard on the nurses, not only as regards training, but also in securing employment after they were trained.[74] The FNA's scheme of training was, apparently, much needed and was taken up with alacrity by a number of hospitals in Britain. The period of grace by which existing fever nurses might register without passing an examination was due to expire in 1911, but it was proposed to extend it for a further year. An examination was due to be held in October 1911 for those who wished to present themselves.[75] Although the FNA's registers have not been traced, the *BJN* is informative, as are two FNA certificates which survive.

The first one, dated 10 July 1911, certifies that 'Miss Agnes Wotherspoon Baird is duly registered by the Fever Nurses' Association as a trained fever nurse', but there is no mention of an examination.[76] Miss Baird trained at the Isolation Hospital, World's End, Winchmore Hill, London under the control of Enfield and Edmonton Joint Hospital Board. Her hospital certificate, dated 28 March 1911, states:

> This is to certify that Agnes Wotherspoon Baird was a nurse in this hospital from 9 January 1909 to 19 February 1911, during which period she received training in Nursing of Patients suffering from Scarlatina, Diphtheria and Enteric Fever. Her conduct and attention to her duties were most satisfactory.[77]

As the period of training is quoted as six weeks in excess of the necessary two years, it is likely that she contracted one or more infectious diseases and had to make up the time when she was off sick.

Before state registration in Britain, it had become custom and practice to issue hospital certificates, testimonials and, in some cases, medals to those who completed courses and passed examinations.[78] A hospital certificate has also been located of a fever nurse who trained at Plaistow Hospital, West Ham, dated 5 April 1915. It states:

> Miss Fanny Elizabeth Ody has received two years Fever training, including Ward instruction and courses of Lectures. She has passed the examinations necessary for this Certificate with credit. Her conduct has been excellent.[79]

The examinations referred to are one set by the Plaistow Hospital, which had been approved for training by the FNA, and the one issued by the FNA (see Appendix 4.1).[80]

A typical examination paper, published in the *BJN* in 1914, indicates the course of instruction that was given in the FNA-approved course. It was taken by fever nurses in London from Plaistow and the MAB Eastern and South Western Hospitals, and nurses from other large institutions in Birmingham, Brighton, Leeds, Newcastle, Paisley, Salford, Sheffield and Southampton.

The following are the questions set by the Fever Nurses' Association for its examination on April 1st [1914].

General Trained Nurses were required to answer only those questions in the Paper which relate to fever and fever nursing.

The time allowed for the Paper was two hours for General Trained Nurses and three hours for Probationers.

### QUESTIONS

1 Give a brief description of the Circulation, including the general, pulmonary, and portal systems.
2 What are the constituents of food? Illustrate your answer by reference to a breakfast consisting of bacon and egg, bread, butter, and coffee.
3 What points would be important in choosing a room in a private house for the isolation and nursing of an infectious case? How would you prepare the isolated quarters?
4 What are the chief signs of danger in Scarlet Fever and its complications? Which of them would lead you to make an immediate report to the Medical Officer in hospital cases?
5 Describe the nursing of a case of Enteric Fever; and mention the more common complications and their chief symptoms.
6 What do you understand by Infectious Material? Whence does the infection come and how is it conveyed in the following diseases: (1) Scarlet Fever; (2) Enteric Fever; (3) Smallpox, and (4) Diphtheria?[81]

*Figure 2.7* Fever Nurses' Association Examination for Certificate of Fever Training, April 1914.

By 1916, it was reported that 2,189 members and nurses held the FNA certificate, some of whom had taken the FNA examinations.[82] This number was relatively small, considering that by 1914 there were 755 isolation hospitals in England and Wales alone (see Table 2.2). It is apparent that many of these hospitals were not approved by the FNA and their nurses could not have received the benefits of the scheme. The main beneficiary seems to have been the large fever hospitals, especially the MAB, which still set its own examinations based on the FNA scheme, and like other fever hospitals, also issued its own certificates.

## Conclusion

During much of the nineteenth century, the primary aim of isolation hospitals was to contain the feverish sick, to separate them from the 'healthy'. Legislation to enable this was slow in Britain, although Ireland passed an Act in 1818 to establish fever hospitals. The wording summed up the contemporary philosophy: attention was to be paid to relieve the suffering poor and, perhaps, more importantly from a national viewpoint, to prevent the increase of infectious fevers in Ireland. Throughout Britain, the condition of the masses was poor and premature death was common. Lack of professional nursing care in the community meant that the only recourse was to a workhouse, which may have had an infirmary or fever ward. Isolation hospitals were only slowly provided on an *ad-hoc* basis and high mortality rates of patients admitted too late did little to enhance their reputation. This in turn led to concealment of the seriously ill. Nursing care, initially, was really guardianship of patients in hospitals, what Goffman refers to in a parallel situation in mental asylums and prisons as 'storage dumps for inmates'.[83] This analogy is particularly apt, as patients were unlikely to receive a reasonable standard of care then because of the primitive nature of early hospitals and the ignorance of the nurses. Even when the number of hospitals increased, the situation did not necessarily improve, because there were insufficient women with knowledge and experience to staff them. Transformation of fever nursing in large institutions was brought about through discipline, training and improved conditions in hospitals and nurses' homes, which attracted a better class of nurse. Nursing care of patients gradually came to be seen as important as their incarceration.

Isolation hospitals did not have the monopoly of caring for patients with infectious diseases as they were to be found in most other institutions. It follows that every nurse really needed to know about them, wherever she was working, a fact which applied just as much to men working as lunatic asylum attendants. As the women who formed the main workforce in isolation hospitals were originally of the servant class, sometimes of ill repute and relatively uneducated, an authoritarian system of management was very necessary. Those who entered fever nursing and demurred against the systems in place were quickly dismissed, or left of their own accord. Doctors, who were usually of a higher social class than the majority of fever nurses, had had a good general and medical education. They were rightly appalled at the low standard of care meted out to patients, but were usually prepared to help matrons, lady superintendents, and in one case in Glasgow, someone who was not a nurse, to improve the situation. By the end of the nineteenth century, they were giving courses of lectures, issuing certificates, writing textbooks for fever nurses and playing a large part in organising and supervising this branch of the profession in most parts of Britain.

This is particularly evident in the foundation of the FNA in 1908. The schemes of fever nurse training it set up – two years for a new probationer, one year for a nurse trained in a general hospital approved by the FNA – were at odds with the three-year course already established in some Scottish hospitals. Neither did it apparently take into account laudable, integrated schemes, whereby probationers in general and children's hospitals were seconded for a three- or six-month period to a fever hospital to gain experience. Nor were small isolation hospitals considered, although they took in young women and referred to them as probationers. The FNA appears to have washed its hands of them, a situation which did not enhance patient care. Nursing care in many large isolation hospitals in Britain had improved by the early twentieth century, but fever nurses, in particular the matrons, were concerned with their professional status and where fever nursing fitted into state registration. Until legislation was enacted, hospital certificates were the main hallmark of a 'good nurse'. As will be seen in the next chapter, other countries were to lead the way in regularising the nursing profession through legislation.

## Notes and references*

1 Searle (1965), p.4.
2 Goffman (1991[1961]), pp. 23–30.
3 Newman (1906), pp. 168–69, and see M. R. Currie (1998) 'Social Policy and Public Health Measures in Bedfordshire, within the National Context, 1904–1938', unpublished PhD thesis, University of Luton, pp. 45–48. George Newman, County MOH, Bedfordshire, 1900–07, became Chief Medical Officer of the Board of Education until 1919, when he took on the additional role of Chief Medical Officer of the newly established Ministry of Health, posts he held until his retirement in 1935.
4 Frazer (1950), p. 121.
5 Hardy (1993), p. 4.
6 Dingwall (2003), p. 169.
7 N. S. Galbraith and J. R. H. Berrie (1978) 'Statutory Notification and Surveillance of Infectious Diseases', *Health Trends*, Part 10, 32–34. Ophthalmia neonatorum, a condition affecting the eyes of neonates, contracted during vaginal delivery from mothers infected with gonorrhoea, was listed in 1914 (see Appendix 1).

*————
Full references appear in the Bibliography.

8 Weeks (1989), pp. 85, 91. See also Bell (1962).

9 Merry and Irven (1960), pp. 6–9. The Queen had received a gift of a large sum of money from the Women's Jubilee Offering of Great Britain and Ireland; of this she donated £70,000 to advance district nursing nationally. The interest from the fund, £2,000 per annum, was used to establish the Queen Victoria Jubilee Institute for Nurses to provide education for nurses to tend the sick poor in their own homes. In 1925, Queen Mary succeeded as patron, and the name was changed to the Queen's Institute of District Nursing. In 1953, Queen Elizabeth, the Queen Mother, became patron. It is now called the Queen's Nursing Institute.

10 Morten (n.d. [1899]), p. 196. Scarletina (scarlet fever) is usually spelt scarlatina.

11 Sworder (1893).

12 Annual Report, MOH, Borough of Luton, 1936, p. 97.

13 Cook, and Stevenson (1988), p. 55.

14 Richardson (1998), pp. 133–34.

15 Cashman (1988), p. 25.

16 Currie (1982), pp. 34, 38.

17 Richardson (1998), p. 1.

18 Ayers (1971), pp. 61–62, 97, 274. See Figure 5 following p. 370. Ayers fails to include the Fountain Hospital (1893) in the list given on p. 274, but does mention it on p. 97 as a makeshift hospital. On p. 276 she gives it erroneously as a mental hospital in 1893. In fact, it was not until 1911 that the MAB removed the Fountain from its Isolation Hospitals' Service and reallocated it as a mental hospital for the treatment of the lowest grade of severely subnormal children. With additions and alterations, this temporary hospital survived until the early 1960s, when it was demolished to make way for the new St George's Hospital, Tooting. Information from English Heritage, 10 October 2003.

19 Burdett (1893), pp. 104–05.

20 K. Maglen (2002) ' "The First Line of Defence": British Quarantine and the Port Sanitary Authorities in the Nineteenth Century', *Social History of Medicine*, 15(3): 413–15.

21 Burdett (1893), vol. IV, p. 280.

22 Annual Report, County MOH, Durham County Council, 1902, pp. xi, 177–79.

23 Taylor (1991), p. 111.

24 Richardson (1998), p. 140. Typical plans are shown on p. 141. In 1919, the Ministry of Health assumed the responsibilities of the LGB.

25 Annual Report, MOH, Borough of Luton, 1936, p. 97.

26 Richardson (1998), p. 140.

27 Ibid., p. 142.

28 G. Cronje (1984) 'Tuberculosis and Mortality Decline in England and Wales, 1851–1910', in Woods and Woodward (1984), pp. 79–80.

29 Lane (2001), p. 143.

30 Abel-Smith (1964), pp. 127–28.

31 Scanlan (1991), pp. 4–5.

32 Ibid., pp. 58, 64.

33 Donnelly (2001), pp. 103, 105.

34 Clarkson and Crawford (2001), p. 4. In their defence, there was total ignorance of the true nature and origins of typhus until 1909, when it was discovered that the body louse was the causative factor. See Hardy (1993), p. 2. The louse also transmitted relapsing fever.

35 Thompson (n.d.) p. 25.

36 McKenzie (2000), p. 52.

37 This comment is quoted verbatim.

38 McKenzie (2000), pp. 54–55, 57–62, 85. Mrs Sinclair was still in post in 1906; she died in 1921.

39 Gray (1999), pp. 7–18.

40 Census of Scotland, 1921.

41 Census of Scotland, 1921 and *Burdett's Hospitals and Charities, 1922–23*. The data given may not be an absolute indicator of population due to different catchment areas.

42 Gray (1999), pp. 156, 354.

43 Royal College of Nursing Archives (RCNA) C69. Rules for the Management of the City Hospital for Infectious Diseases at Walker Gate, City and County of Newcastle upon Tyne, April 1909.

44 Ayers (1971), pp. 23, 147.

45 LGB (1882) Tenth Annual Report of the Local Government Board 1880–81, *C3290 Use and Influence of Hospitals for Infectious Diseases*, London: HMSO.

46 Gray (1999), p. 58.

47 *Burdett's Hospitals and Charities, 1899*.

48 C. Maggs (1981) 'The Register of Nurses in the Scottish Poor Law Service 1885–1919', *Nursing Times*, 25 November: 129–30. This 'occasional paper' is key to the understanding of the development of nursing in Scotland.

49 Ibid: 130–31.

50 Scanlan (1991), p. 82.

51 The National Library of Ireland, Dublin (NLI). 'Lady Superintendents of the Irish Hospitals', *The Lady of the House*, Christmas 1902, p. 27. A photograph of Miss Carson Rae is included in this special edition.

52 NLI. 'The Nurses of the Irish Hospitals, No. VIII – Nursing School of Cork Street Fever Hospital', *The Lady of the House*, 15 June 1895, p. 3. The proper title for Jervis Street Hospital is the Charitable Infirmary, Jervis Street.

53 London Metropolitan Archives, LMA 1228 Nursing Staff Committee Minutes, 9 June 1893 - 10 February 1899, p. 76.

54 Royal Free Hospital Archive/London Fever Hospital (RFHA/LFH) 1/HD/1/3. London Fever Hospital, House Directors Minutes, 1878–83.

55 LMA 1228 MAB Nursing Staff Committee Minutes 9 June 1893 – 10 February 1899, between pp. 102–03.

56 Ayers (1971), p. 150.

57 LMA H9/GY/C4/2, Matron's Journal 1901–05, Guy's Hospital.

58 RFHA, North Western Fever Hospital 2/2, Register of Officers: Nursing Staff Register 1904–11 (Book 1).

59 Archives of the Faculty of Nursing and Midwifery, Royal College of Surgeons in Ireland, Dublin. Minutes of Proceedings of the Governing Authority, Dublin Metropolitan Technical School for Nurses (DMTSN), 16 December 1893, cited in McGann (1992), p. 136; the author includes a whole section on the DMTSN, pp. 135–36. Cork Street Fever Hospital also availed itself of the programme of lectures offered by the DMTSN (information from Dr Gerard Fealy, University College Dublin, 8 January 2004).

60 RCNA. M. Donaldson (1983) 'The Development of Nursing in Northern Ireland', unpublished DPhil thesis, New University of Ulster, p. 48.

61 Ibid., pp. 358, 363. Following the Nurses Registration (Ireland) Act, 1919, it was the only hospital approved for training for the Fever Register by the Joint Nursing and Midwives Council for Northern Ireland.

62 A. K. Gordon (1907) 'The Position of the Isolation Hospital in the Training of a Nurse', *British Journal of Nursing*, 26 January: 63–65. Dr Gordon was previously a MAB assistant medical officer, and later Medical Superintendent of Monsall Fever Hospital, Manchester.

63 *BJN*, 2 February 1907: 81–2.

64 *BJN*, 8 June 1907: 421.

65 Ibid: 437–8.

66 *BJN*, 15 June 1907: 457.

67 The *BJN*, previously the *Nursing Record* (1888–1902), was bought by Dr Bedford Fenwick for his wife in 1899. Her influence and views pervade these journals. She died in 1947; the *BJN* ceased publication in 1956.

68 *BJN*, 25 January 1908: 70.

69 *BJN*, 11 July 1908: 30–31. Dr Goodall became the Honorary Medical Secretary of the Central Committee for the State Registration of Nurses from 1910. For more detailed information about Susan Villiers, see entry in *Oxford Dictionary of National Biography* (Oxford: Oxford University Press, 2004). Chapter 7 in this book is devoted to her and Harriet Cassells.

70 Ibid.

71 LMA MAB 26.03, Board Minutes 1909, vol. XLIII, 19–20 and 163. A copy of the Syllabus of Lectures was published in the *BJN*, 21 August 1909: 158.

72 *BJN*, 29 May 1909: 431.

73 King's College London Archives, Royal British Nurses' Association (KCLA/RBNA), GB0099. Administrative/Biographical History. The Association was renamed the Royal BNA in 1891 and received its Royal Charter in 1893.

74 M. Drakard (1910) 'The Nurse in Fever Hospitals', *Nursing Times*, 5 November: 906.

75 *BJN*, 27 May 1911: 414.

76 KCLA/RBNA/P172/79. FNA certificate no. 1031, Agnes Wotherspoon Baird, 10 July 1911. This certificate is in a poor state of preservation.

77 KCLA/RBNA/P172/80. Hospital certificate of Agnes Wotherspoon Baird, 28 March 1911.

78 Even after state registration, most hospitals continued to conduct their own examinations, award certificates and hospital badges and sometimes medals, but testimonials, which could be forged, were seldom issued after the Second World War (1939–45).

79 RCNA C148/1 Hospital certificate, Fanny Elizabeth Ody, 5 April 1915.

80 RCNA, C148/2 FNA certificate no. 1929, Fanny Elizabeth Ody, 6 April 1915.

81 *BJN*, 23 May 1914: 462.

82 *BJN*, 24 June 1916: 550.

83 Goffman (1991[1961]), p. 73.

# 3 State registration to the decline of fever nursing

Unless a nurse is encouraged to proceed fairly soon [from fever training] to her general training, she loses her enthusiasm . . . and remains a partially trained woman, whose value in the future will be less and less, as I feel sure that most posts which are worth having will go to registered nurses.

Susan Villiers (1925)[1]

## Introduction

Professional fever nursing was slow to evolve in Britain, but towards the end of the nineteenth century, capable general trained nurses began to take the lead as matrons or nurse superintendents in large isolation hospitals, although they were not fever trained, as it scarcely existed then. They established training schools, based on the same rigorous standards they had experienced in their own general training, where they would, almost certainly, have nursed patients with infectious diseases. Since the 1880s, such women were beginning to consider whether nurses should be tested by public examination and have a register set up, with the title 'nurse' restricted to duly registered candidates. Doctors had already achieved statutory registration under the Medical Act, 1858.[2]

The concept of state registration for nurses proved to be an extremely controversial professional issue, partly because two of the most influential British nurses, Florence Nightingale (1820–1910) and Mrs Bedford Fenwick (1857–1947) held opposing views. Fever nurse leaders were involved in the sometimes acrimonious debates which eventually led to the state registration of fever nurses. Decisions made in the period following 1919 were to have international repercussions. As this chapter covers a number of important issues, a chronological approach has been adopted for each, of which state registration is the most important.

## Progress towards state registration: international influences

Mrs Fenwick (née Ethel Gordon Manson, Matron of St Bartholomew's Hospital, London, 1881–87) was the leader of the pro-registration faction, ably supported by her new husband, Dr Bedford Fenwick, a well-known physician. In 1887, they set up a meeting at their house in London, of nurses 'whose aims were the control of nursing by Act of Parliament', at which the British Nurses' Association was established. Dr Fenwick cajoled the British Medical Association into passing a resolution in favour of the registration of nurses and, in 1889, a mass meeting at the Mansion House called for an official register of nurses. Florence Nightingale's opposition was partly because she believed that a central examination could undermine her whole philosophy about nursing, which emphasised the right personal qualities and aptitudes. 'Nursing has to do with living spirits and bodies. It cannot be tested by public examination, though it may be tested by current supervision'.[3]

The ever resourceful Mrs Fenwick was a keen and outspoken supporter of women's rights. She constantly sought new ways to promote her cause for registration through the Matrons' Council of Great Britain and Ireland, which she founded in 1894, and at the International Council of Women, which met in London in 1899, at which the Matrons' Council began campaigning for an International Council of Nurses. The new organisation was duly established and held its first Congress in Buffalo, New York State, in 1901, with Mrs Fenwick as its first president. She reiterated her theme, that 'the nurse question was the Woman Question' and that 'our profession, like every other profession, needs registration'.[4] At that time, there was little mention of separate registers for fever nurses or other specialist branches.

Since most countries in the British Empire were not then involved in internal professional wrangles, it is probable that they were freer to enact legislation earlier than in Britain. In New Zealand, the Nurses Registration Act, 1901, was passed on 12 September and came into force on 1 January 1902, when the Register of Nurses was set up. The first nurses whose names were entered had trained at various hospitals in Britain and New Zealand, so the precedent for reciprocity was established. However, there was not a section for fever nurses then or later when separate registers were developed. Midwifery was always a separate discipline and was recognised professionally following the Midwives Act, 1904,[5] two years later than the Midwives Act, 1902 in England and Wales. Although South Africa sometimes claims to have been the first to have state registration in 1891, it was actually embedded in an Act relating to medicine. New Zealand was, therefore, the first country to have separate legislation for nursing registration.[6]

In the late nineteenth century, hospital authorities in the United States began to recognise the advantages of having 'a ready supply of inexpensive labor'. New hospitals and 'sanitariums' [*sic*] were established and 400 nurse training schools were incorporated into these institutions. Between 1890 and 1902, momentum gathered for registration and separate state associations were formed to implement strategies to achieve legal regulation. North Carolina was the first state to enact a registration law in 1903, followed by New Jersey, New York and Virginia in the same year. Twenty years later, legislation to regulate nursing was operative in 48 states.[7] However,

Sub types or special programs for nurses did not appear in the US. Instead, there was a strong drive for standardization beginning in the mid 1890s – efforts to develop distinct programs were discouraged – although insane asylums and tuberculosis hospitals did open training schools they usually argued that their programs prepared for general practice. Thus specialized practice was built on the basic program either through experience or short training programs – examples of this would be nurse anesthesia and public health.[8]

It seems, therefore, that the development of fever nursing as a specialism was peculiar to Britain.

## Delayed state registration in Britain

Dr and Mrs Fenwick founded the Society for the State Registration of Nurses in 1902, which drafted the first Bill for state registration in 1903; it was introduced into Parliament in 1904, but met fierce opposition and was defeated. The Royal British Nurses' Association promoted a separate Bill in 1904. As a result of strong feelings within the House of Commons and the nursing profession, a House of Commons Select Committee on the registration of nurses was appointed that same year.[9] The Committee reported in favour of state registration in 1905. The pro-registrationists were convinced that state regulation of their profession could no longer be postponed, but the Bills introduced in the House of Commons in 1906 and 1907, by private members, lacked government support and were blocked by their opponents.[10] This political activity took place in London, but other parts of the profession in Britain did not necessarily approve of decisions made there which might not take their needs into account.

The movement to create a system of state registration had really begun in Scotland in 1885, when 'an excellent system of certification' was introduced in poorhouses by the Local Government Board for Scotland. It merely needed developing into a 'system of statutory regulation'. However, in March 1909, some Scottish medical men called a meeting in Glasgow. They opposed Lord Ampthill's Bill, because it proposed that there should not be a separate Nursing Council for Scotland. This would leave Scottish nurses with practically no representation under a Registration Council which had its headquarters in London. Their main concern was to ensure reciprocity with branch councils in England and Ireland. 'Nurses registered in Scotland must be acceptable as nurses registered in England, not only within the boundaries of the British Isles but in the colonies as well'. Following the meeting, an Association for the Promotion of Registration in Scotland was formed, with a committee of leading medical men and matrons.[11]

The possibility of a successful passage through Parliament of a nurses' registration Act was delayed, therefore, for professional, and political reasons, including time spent on considerable debate about campaigns by militant suffragettes, and the quieter reasonings of the suffragists and others desirous of obtaining 'Votes for Women'. Another time-consuming issue was the 'Irish Question'. Home Rule for Ireland was sought, which would give partial self-government and the re-creation of an Irish Parliament.[12] Unsuccessful Home Rule Bills were introduced in 1886 and 1893. In 1914, Irish Home Rule and State Registration were delayed still further by the outbreak of the First World War.[13]

During this war, the Fever Nurses' Association became involved in other controversies affecting the nursing profession, including the proposed establishment of a new College of Nursing. The Central Committee for the State Registration of Nurses (CCSRN) on which the FNA was represented, had drafted the latest Nurse Registration Bill, yet the FNA had not been consulted about the establishment of the new college. This was particularly inflammatory, as it was suggested that the college should undertake many of the duties and functions of the proposed General Nursing Council (GNC), including those the FNA had previously performed.[14] Even before this, in 1912, Lavinia Dock, the American nurse historian, observed that:

> The hospital world of England was divided into two camps. The progressives had as their goal the organisation of nurses through a central government body appointed by the State ... the reactionaries would not admit the necessity for fixing a minimum standard of training and were strongly averse to organisation amongst nurses ... For twenty-three years the battle was waged, and is not yet ended.
>
> (*A History of Nursing*, vol. III, pp. 33–34)[15]

In English terms, the progressives were known as pro-registrationists or registrationists and the reactionaries as anti-registrationists; in this context, resolution was difficult. However, as previously mentioned, Scotland had already made tremendous advances in the professionalisation of nurses. In 1911, the LGB for Scotland introduced a Fever Nurse Certificate to make training more uniform in the 'great fever hospitals'. Not only did the fever nurse receive a hospital certificate, but one provided by the state and a badge, white on blue enamelled saltire, surrounded by silver lettering, 'REGISTERED FEVER NURSE, SCOTLAND'.[16] Long lists of names of successful candidates who now possessed the LGB fever certificate of efficiency were published in the *British Journal of Nursing*.[17]

Ireland was also, it appears, tired of waiting for decisive action in Parliament in London, and considered how the professional interests of Irish nurses, including fever nurses, could best be met. It seems that disillusionment with nursing organisations elsewhere in Britain set in during the First World War. For example, when the College of Nursing was established in London in 1916, it had an elected Council of thirty-six members, which included six representatives from Ireland. At that time, Ireland was vigorously attempting to obtain freedom from Britain, so the idea of an association with it, did not appeal to Irish nurses. In 1917 an Irish Nursing Board was formed to establish a register of all trained nurses in Ireland and to develop a 'proper standard of nursing education'. The new Board comprised four doctors, elected by the College of Surgeons and twenty-two nurses.[18]

## State registration in Britain

In November 1918, the First World War came to an end; the government could now turn to other matters. In November 1919, the new Minister of Health, Dr Addison, exasperated by the internal politics within the nursing profession, urged the withdrawal of two State Registration Bills and put forward his own Bill. As there were three Ministries of Health, three Registration Acts were necessary which would provide three separate GNCs, hence, the Nurses Registration (England and Wales) Act, 1919, the Nurses Registration (Scotland) Act, 1919, and the Nurses Registration (Ireland) Act, 1919. However, it was only following last-minute lobbying by the Irish pro-registration movement that analogous Irish registration legislation was enacted. A deputation representing the Irish Nurses' Association, the Irish Matrons' Association and the Irish Board had travelled to Westminster to lobby for the introduction of an Irish registration bill in early November 1919, as the Irish nursing world was alarmed that Ireland was not included in Dr Addison's Bill. The Bills received the Royal Assent and became law throughout the British Isles on 23 December 1919.[19] Having achieved state registration, the nursing profession had to overcome a number of anomalies concerning the duration of training and reciprocity, without further examination, not just among the constituent parts of the United Kingdom, but also with other countries.

The new Regulatory Authorities for England and Wales, Scotland and Ireland wanted to continue their established systems of fever nurse training and agreement between them proved difficult. The 'Irish Question' made it even more complex. The Irish War of Independence was ongoing when the GNC for Ireland was being formed in 1920. The Treaty of 1921 ended hostilities and resulted in the establishment of the Irish Free State and the establishment of Northern Ireland as a separate jurisdiction. In this connection, a new and separate regulatory body for nursing and midwifery was constituted, the Joint Nursing and Midwives Council for Northern Ireland (JNMCNI) under the Joint Nursing and Midwives Council Act (Northern Ireland), 1922.[20] The new GNC for Ireland was left with responsibility for professional regulation of nurses in the Irish Free State and, ultimately, to the Minister for Local Government. The Irish Free State comprised twenty-six counties, including three in the province of Ulster. Northern Ireland comprised the remaining six counties: Fermanagh, Antrim, Tyrone, Leitrim, Armagh and Derry (Londonderry).[21]

The new GNC for England and Wales was required to establish and maintain a Register of Nurses that was to have six parts. The first was a general part, then five supplementary parts: for male nurses, mental nurses, nurses of mental defectives, sick children's nurses, and fever nurses, who would, after qualification, become registered fever nurses (RFNs). The general and all supplementary registers, except fever nursing, required a three-year course in an institution approved by the GNC, which decided that the minimum age to register should be 21 years and evidence of good character should be provided.[22] Brian Abel-Smith pointed out forty years later that the General Register had the highest status.[23]

Anne Marie Rafferty's work on the background to the supplementary registers by the GNC for England and Wales reveals further dissension. The aspirations of a broad generalist approach to nurse training went back to 'the original mission of nineteenth century nursing for the reconstruction of social discipline on hygienic principles', but this ideal had always been compromised by the demand for labour by different types of hospitals and the medical profession's need for a skilled, yet subordinate class of labour. The Bedford Fenwick faction, however, attached great importance to the notion of a common entry route for all types of nurses and the concept of supplementary registers for specialists, such as fever nurses, was a complete anathema to them and was derided by the secretary of the RBNA, Isabel McDonald.[24]

The so-called specialists were disparaged as they were regarded as 'semi-educated and unduly susceptible to medical domination'. Mrs Fenwick's antipathy went back to earlier in the century when she opposed the separate licensing of midwives, in much the same way as the medical profession's contempt for groups like the lithotomists, whose practice was not founded on a general training. She was not against 'the medical model of professional organization, but medical intervention in the government of nursing'. However, the caretaker council (nominated by the Minister of Health) was under pressure to produce a registration scheme inclusive of all types of nursing. Although it had managed to agree on one criterion, an initial one-year training in an approved hospital, Mrs Fenwick, who chaired the subcommittee which vetted applications for the register, obstructed progress to such an extent that the majority of members submitted their resignations. It was only an assurance of ministerial support and the threat that the minister would amend the Act, that progress continued. As Mrs Fenwick was defeated in the first council election, her obstruction to the supplementary registers was removed.[25] Agreement over reciprocity was to prove equally contentious.

The issue of reciprocity was particularly difficult for Scotland, as both the general and fever training courses in most large hospitals were one year longer than those in England and Wales, and Ireland. It soon emerged that Scotland intended to maintain the *status quo*, as following the introduction of the LGB fever nurse certificate in 1911, trained fever nurses in Scotland had already gained the RFN qualification. Matrons of most large fever hospitals in Scotland were convinced that their three-year system was the optimum time necessary for a fever nurse course. The new Scottish Health Board (the equivalent of the new Ministry of Health for England and Wales), which replaced the LGB in Scotland in 1919, issued its first certificates to twenty-nine fever nurses in 1920.[26] One of the first to receive this certificate was Catherine Bruce Samuel, who entered fever nurse training at the City Hospital, Edinburgh in September 1917, aged 25 years. She successfully completed her three-year course in September 1920, and therefore received both a hospital and a state certificate (see Appendix 4.2 for her Scottish Board of Health Fever Nurse Certificate).[27] The issue of reciprocity with Scotland concerned the nursing profession in Britain and abroad, Parliament and eminent nurse leaders.

Mrs Fenwick, the first person to have her name entered in the General Register for Nurses in England and Wales, was not a fever nurse, although she usually championed their causes. On 7 July 1921, she convened a meeting with the Minister of Health at the House of Commons on behalf of the RBNA. She had assembled a formidable array of nurse leaders to reinforce the minister's decision to keep to a two-year fever course throughout Britain, and not to accede to Scotland's intention to place general and fever nurses on the same General Register. They included representatives of the Matron's Council of Great Britain and Ireland, the Registered Nurses' Parliamentary Council, the National Union of Trained Nurses, the College of Nursing, Ltd, and the Professional Union of Trained Nurses. The account begins:

> Mrs Bedford Fenwick had the honour to introduce to the Minister of Health a Deputation to protest against the proposal of the Scottish Board of Health to place on the General Register nurses trained in Fever Nursing only. In view of the reciprocity clause in the English, Scottish and Irish Acts, this proposal was not only unfair to the interests of nurses on the General Register, but to English Fever Trained nurses as well . . . The result of this deputation was entirely satisfactory.[28]

In 1921, the GNC for Scotland stated that it had accepted thirteen of the twenty fever nurse applications for registration from 'existing nurses' and 'Nurses in Training before issue of Rules'. It then reported briefly, concealing its displeasure about being defeated at the House of Commons. It was unable to adjust with the GNCs for England and Wales and for Ireland 'The terms on which Nurses registered by the one Council should be re-registered by another Council'.[29] It had still not reached agreement regarding reciprocity in 1922, but had approved combined training schemes in Edinburgh between Chalmers Hospital and the City Fever Hospital.[30] At a meeting of the Education and Examinations Committee of the GNC for England and Wales on 27 February 1923, the matter of reciprocity with Scotland was discussed. Dr Goodall

> Pointed out that he did not think it likely from what he had gathered from correspondence, that Scotland would give way on the three years'

training for the Supplementary Register, and that they were supported by the Society of Medical Officers of Health for Scotland. He asked that the Rules of the General Nursing Council for England and Wales should be approved by the Minister and that there should be no reciprocity between England and Scotland.[31]

This was not in the best interests of fever nurses, who might want to take up employment in a country, other than where they trained. However, the previous systems for fever training in Scotland were doomed as, later that year, the Society of Medical Officers of Health in Scotland represented to the Council, through the Scottish Board of Health, their revised opinion that, 'the period of training for Fever Nurses should be reduced from three to two years'. The Scottish GNC accepted the suggestion and prepared Draft Rules providing for this.[32] Matrons of fever hospitals and some doctors in Scotland were amazed at the GNC's decision to adopt a two-year standard for fever nurse training and found themselves unable to accept it. Matrons said they could not undertake to teach a nurse everything necessary in two years. The matron of one large hospital stated that in spite of the Council's decision, she would continue to train her nurses for three years and took them on that understanding from the beginning.[33] In fact, the third year became a period in which junior staff nurses could consolidate their experience. It also entitled them to their prized hospital certificate (see Appendix 4.9).

Scotland had lost the battle regarding the official duration of training, but it was a Pyrrhic victory regarding the placement of names on the same register. Whereas in England and Wales, separate registers were kept for fever and general nurses, in Scotland the professional register for all branches was maintained in the same volumes with names entered chronologically, with only letters of the alphabet to denote the specialist branch. For example, the prefix 'E' denoted a fever nurse, but the acronym 'EN' meant 'existing nurse' (at the time of state registration). In April 1924, the GNC for Scotland held its first preliminary examination, the same for entry to all branches of nursing. The subjects were Anatomy and Physiology, Hygiene and Elementary Theory and Practice of Nursing, Part I. None of the 73 entrants passed all three parts.[34] The first Final examination was held in October 1925. Nurses who produced a certificate of not less than three years' training by 30 September 1925 were eligible as Intermediate Nurses, but there were relatively few entries. Of the 31 Fever Nurse candidates, 28 passed the First Paper (Infectious Diseases) and 25 passed the Second Paper (Nursing and Cooking).[35]

It is significant that the JNMCNI also segregated different forms of nurse training in the register by a key number. General nursing was accorded the prime place. For example, Harriet May Thompson's Certificate of Registration as a general nurse in 1949 is recorded as A5005, whereas her Certificate as a registered fever nurse in 1947 is number E644 (see Appendix 4.8).

The GNC for Ireland established a register of general nurses and supplementary parts for male nurses, mental nurses, sick children's nurses and a

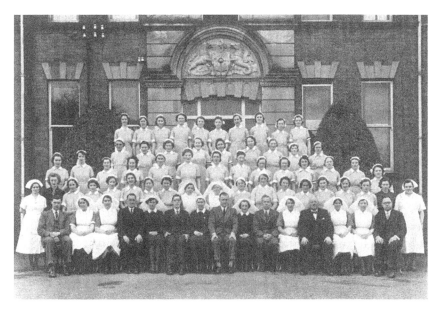

*Figure 3.1* Nursing and medical staff, Purdysburn Fever Hospital, Belfast, 1940.
Courtesy of Mrs Margaret Gorman

register for 'Nurses trained in the Nursing of persons suffering from Infectious Diseases'.[36] Hence, the professional qualification became registered infectious diseases nurse (RIDN), not RFN. Three nurses were entered in 1921, the first year for which the Register of RIDNs was kept; two were entered as 'existing nurses' and one as 'interim'. All had been trained at Cork Street Fever Hospital, Dublin, in the south inner city. By then, Cork Street and the Hardwicke Fever Hospital, in the north inner city, were the principal fever hospitals in Dublin. A further twelve names of nurses were added to the Register in 1922, the majority of whom trained at Cork Street. Other hospitals listed that year, which were also training institutions, were the District Hospital, Cork, the Galway Fever Hospital and the Purdysburn Fever Hospital, Belfast (Figure 3.1). Some of the first nurses were approved through reciprocity, having trained at an approved hospital elsewhere, namely the MAB North Eastern Hospital, London, the City Fever Hospital, Birmingham and Pennsylvania Fever Hospital in the United States.[37]

At the beginning of 1924, there were 2,373 nurses on the general register and 633 mental nurses, 16 sick children's nurses and 18 fever nurses on the supplementary registers.[38] The original grounds for admission to the register were listed as 'existing', 'interim' or 'after examination'. After 1924, the majority of candidates admitted to all parts of the register were 'after examination'.[39] The Nurses Act, 1950, dissolved the GNC for Ireland and the Central Midwives Board, and the new Nursing Board (An Bord Altranais) was established to regulate nursing and midwifery in the Irish Republic.

There were 1,176 names entered on the Register for RIDNs in Ireland between 1921 and 1950; most nurses had undertaken the full two-year course.[40] Nurses who had already undergone a three-year basic course in general or children's nursing were able to take a one-year training programme. By the early 1960s, 25 nurses annually undertook this course at Cherry Orchard Fever Hospital (previously Dublin Fever Hospital). The oral and written examinations included knowledge of nursing, fevers and bacteriology and infectious diseases (see Appendix 4.10).[41] This hospital was still carrying out the full two-year programme as late as 1964.[42]

At the GNC for England and Wales, the interests of fever nurses were represented on both the Caretaker Council, 1920–22, and the first Elected Council, 1923–27, by Miss Villiers (FNA), who was elected to the Finance and the Education and Examinations Committees. As a consequence, the FNA 'came to an end' in 1926.[43] The names of nurses continued to be registered in the Scottish Register of Sick Nurses and in the separate one for fever nurses until 1930, although the system of examinations was taken over by the Scottish GNC prior to that date.[44]

## The inter-war years

At the annual meeting of the FNA on 23 May, 1925, Susan Villiers, Matron of the MAB South Western Hospital, Stockwell, and a member of the GNC for England and Wales, took the chair. In her wide-ranging presidential address she noted that much of the work formerly undertaken by the association was now being carried out by the GNC. She paid tribute to the early work of the FNA, which had standardised the training of fever nurses, and to Dr John Biernacki, the founder of the FNA. Miss Villiers then raised the issue of establishing preliminary training schools (PTSs). She endorsed the issue of affiliating fever hospitals with general hospitals, which would result in general and fever trained nurses, for unless a fever trained nurse proceeded fairly soon to general training, Miss Villiers felt that she would remain 'a partially-trained woman'. She was also concerned that, in epidemics, girls of a lower standard of education had to be engaged. More trained nurses could be employed, or temporary assistant nurses engaged, but these women should not be kept so long that they considered themselves equal to certificated fever nurses.[45]

At the same meeting, Dr Caiger, the honorary treasurer, presented a balance sheet which showed that £362 14s 2d (£362.71) was in hand at the end of the financial year, £250 of which had been placed on deposit. He reminded members that the income would not be so large in the future as the FNA examinations had ceased in April that year (1925), and the fees from these were their main source of income. Regarding the future status and functions of the association, as a medical man he believed that now that the functions had been so largely assumed by the GNC, it might be prudent to reconstitute the association with the lady members carrying it forward. He also expressed deep regret at the death of Miss Isla Stewart (Matron of St Bartholomew's Hospital 1887–1910) in 1910 as, had she lived, he believed she would have been instrumental in establishing a system of reciprocal training between fever and general hospitals.[46] The outcome of the 1925 meeting was that a League of Fever Nurses was established.

Among the many responsibilities with which the new GNCs were involved, which required different committees, was the mammoth task of inspecting fever hospitals for approval for fever nurse training. As the experience of FNA nurse leaders had been gained in large isolation hospitals, including those run by the MAB, they were likely to be biased in favour of large hospitals. They were unlikely, therefore, to approve the limited form of fever nurse training possible in much smaller, and less busy, institutions. The system set up by the FNA in 1909 provided a model scheme for large hospitals, not just for the MAB but for the GNC for England and Wales. Because of the large number and the sheer size of some hospitals, only those considered doubtful were inspected. From the inception of the FNA in 1908, matrons and medical superintendents of fever hospitals worked together for a common cause (see Appendix 2). This may not have been for purely altruistic reasons; the matrons were glad of professional advice from their medical colleagues, while they needed an obedient, but intelligent, workforce to carry out their orders and sometimes to use their own initiative. Training courses were the means by which this could be provided. GNC approval was, therefore, eagerly sought by large and small hospitals, not all of whom operated to the standards laid down by the GNC.

Two hospitals, in particular, were in dispute about standards which the GNC for England and Wales demanded. For example, Darlington Infectious Diseases Hospital operated a three-year system for probationers, but the GNC could not recognise the third year. A letter was sent to the Ministry of Health from Mr H. Hopkins, the Town Clerk of Darlington on 6 July 1925, defending the third year on a number of grounds. For instance, certain duties were regarded as only suitable for a probationer; ward maids would not carry them out and 'it is not customary for trained nurses . . . nor will they do them without protest'. Moreover, some girls had refused to come to the hospital as probationers once they found that it was not recognised for training. This meant that if probationers could not be obtained, the Corporation would have to provide more trained nurses. The hospital operated the same curriculum as the FNA, identical to that laid down by the GNC. In an undated letter, signed 'Brock', to the Right Hon. Neville Chamberlain (Minister of Health), Hopkins explained that the hospital could accommodate 128 patients, including 23 for the isolation of smallpox. The range of infectious diseases was less than in a larger hospital, being mainly confined to scarlet fever and diphtheria, but more experience could be gained during the third year of training. An appeal by Darlington Corporation was held on 25 November 1925, which was granted on 24 February 1926.[47]

Another dispute concerned Hastings Infectious Diseases Hospital, which the GNC had refused to approve as a complete training school for fever nurses because it had fewer than 100 beds. A considerable correspondence on the matter was exchanged between the GNC, the County Borough of Hastings and the Ministry of Health between September 1926 and December 1927. The hospital was eventually approved, although in future it would have to run a course of three years in order to provide sufficient experience for training. The GNC felt aggrieved at the minister's decision to overrule them, yet again. Miss Elaine Musson, Chairman of the Council, wrote on 14 June 1927, that:

> smaller infectious diseases hospitals could never become efficient train-ing schools . . . they only did so because probationers were cheap . . . if the local authorities agreed on the common policy they could quite easily ignore the Council and the Register.[48]

The GNC passed a resolution at the meeting on 18 November 1927, strongly protesting against the minister's decision as, 'it not only permits totally insufficient training in this particular hospital, but will by its effect prevent an adequate standard from being maintained'. Although the GNC appealed about the minister's decision on 15 March 1927, it did not succeed.[49]

During the 1930s, the main problem for fever hospitals was attracting enough probationers. It was only by reducing the age of entry for training to 17 years that wards could be staffed. The GNCs issued criteria to ensure standards were maintained, but as was seen, they could be overruled by central government. The criteria demanded that sufficient training material (patients with a range of infectious diseases) be available to ensure a variety of experience for every probationer. Educational facilities should include systematic arrangements to ensure every probationer was able to attend a series of lectures on prescribed subjects. For training in fever nursing in a complete training school, the requisite period was not less than two years (see Appendix 4.4).

When a fever hospital did not have sufficient material to become a complete school it could be affiliated to one that satisfied the criteria; the period of training would then be extended to two and a half years. Provision was also made for a four-year course in general and fever nurse training, with two years' training in an approved complete training school for fever nurses, followed by two years in an approved complete training school for general nurses. Alternatively, three years' training could be carried out in a complete training school for general nurses and one year subsequently in a complete training school for fever nurses.[50] Clearly, the GNCs had taken notice of earlier schemes; all combinations were covered to maximise opportunities and attract the greatest number of probationers. Although discussion may have taken place about admitting men to training before the Second World War, it does not appear to have been documented.

## Men in fever nursing

Monks and friars are known to have played an important caring role in medieval hospitals, but following the dissolution of the monasteries in the sixteenth century, men seldom appear in parish records caring for patients with fevers in the community. As isolation hospitals became established, there were some opportunities. The MAB in London recognised their worth when the Board's hospital at Deptford was opened for male smallpox patients during the period 1876–78. Due to the shortage of women, the wards were staffed entirely by men. The medical superintendent later affirmed that the men were far preferable to women as ward attendants, despite the extra vigilance required from medical officers during the early stages of the disease. The patients were from the lowest class of the population and the male staff were 'better fitted to maintain order'.[51]

Matrons in fever hospitals had a caring role for their probationers, most of whom were young women under the age of majority. Since matrons were *in loco parentis*, men were perceived as a threat. The apparent hidden agenda about accepting men for fever nurse training was at last overcome in the years following the Second World War. One practical reason for the delay may have been the type of residential accommodation available for probationers. Some small hospitals provided only cubicles; separate rooms were not allocated until after qualification, and nurses' homes were a totally female preserve. Brian Abel-Smith attributes the prejudice against men in nursing to feminism, snobbery and probably 'deeper sexual taboos'. Possibly, male nurses would prove harder to order around, or they might upset the chastity thought appropriate for females 'called' to nursing or, worse still, some even might prove to be homosexual. Moreover, Abel Smith considers that when women obtained power, they used it to discriminate against men. When the new GNC registers were established in England and Wales, male nurses were not admitted to the most prestigious general register.[52]

It was not until the Nurses Act, 1949, that 'the part of the Register for Male Nurses' was closed. The GNC was also given the power to close other parts.[53] Male nurses were not admitted to membership of the Royal College of Nursing until 1960, but neither were student nurses, nor other nurses on the supplementary registers, including fever nurses. In 1937, the Trades Union Congress (TUC), was incensed with the RCN for opposing a bill presented to Parliament for calling for the immediate introduction of a 48 hour week for nurses. In its onslaught on the RCN, the TUC called it 'an organisation of voluntary snobs', that is an organisation which represented the voluntary hospitals, not the municipal hospitals.[54] This retort certainly applied to fever nurses as much as those in public assistance institutions and men. As a result of these rebuffs, many men felt more comfortable and effective in mental nursing, public assistance infirmaries, occupational health work and, increasingly, nurse education.

The first Fever Nurse Syllabus issued by the GNC for England and Wales in 1923 stated that:

> The two years' sojourn in the fever hospital, with studies wisely directed and opportunities happily seized, should prove an excellent entrance to a nurse's career, and should render easier for her the course she takes up later at the general hospital.[55]

Men were excluded by the GNC; they did not have equal opportunities with women, but attitudes towards male fever nurse probationers began to change in the 1940s, as during the war some servicemen gained nursing experience as medical orderlies in isolation hospitals, while others sought a change of career. Their acceptance into fever nurse training in the post war period now gave them parity with female nurses, should they wish to go on to general nurse training, or use their fever nurse training as a second qualification. Nevertheless, in 1954, the GNC for England and Wales still defined 'fever nurses' in terms of female pronouns in the documents they issued: 'A candidate presenting herself for the Final Examination' (Figures 3.2 and 3.3).[56] Not surprisingly, male fever nurses were few and far between. The name of the first male fever nurse was recorded in the supplementary Fever Nurse Register in England and Wales on 23 July 1948.[57] He was one of eight male fever nurses registered between the beginning of 1948 and June 1949, when there were fifty-seven male students in training.[58] None is recorded in the Register of Infectious Diseases Nurses in the Irish Republic.[59] Isolation hospitals were provided with an alternative source of labour in the post-war period, but few availed themselves of the opportunity. Nevertheless, the men who persisted and gained a qualification in the speciality, reinforced with general or mental training, found that it gave them an invaluable springboard into a worthwhile career.

## Health risks to fever nurses

Working in an isolation hospital had always been hazardous and this may be one of the reasons why recruitment was difficult. Before the advances made in bacteriology in the 1880s, it had long been known that a person in direct contact with, or in the near vicinity of, someone with a fever, was likely to contract the disease, even if the route of transmission was not always clearly understood. Patients admitted to a fever hospital with one infectious disease, frequently contracted another while they were there, and women who entered fever nursing, or nursed fever patients elsewhere, were liable to become ill from the same diseases as their patients. In 1900, George Newman, County MOH for Bedfordshire, wrote: 'Only persons beyond middle age should act as nurses to typhoid cases'.[60]

The older a probationer was on entry to training, the less likely she was to become infected, as by then she had probably already had most common childhood diseases, such as measles and scarlet fever. The use of rubber gloves was a rare preventive measure in fever nursing in the early twentieth century, yet by 1902, nurses at Monsall Hospital, Manchester, were using them in the enteric (typhoid) wards, with 'a marked diminution in the incidence of enteric fever amongst staff'.[61] Gradually, nurses learned the wisdom of preventive measures, but there were times when they deliberately put themselves at risk, for example, by volunteering to nurse smallpox patients or by carrying out hazardous procedures. In 1910, Miss Annie Peck,

THE GENERAL NURSING COUNCIL FOR ENGLAND AND WALES.

The Board of Examiners by whom this paper was set is constituted as follows:—
E. JAMES, Esq., M.D., D.P.H.                    MISS J. BLUNT, S.R.N., R.F.N.
W. GUNN, Esq., M.A., M.R.C.P., D.P.H.           MISS E. C. WHITE, S.R.N., R.F.N.

FINAL STATE EXAMINATION FOR THE SUPPLEMENTARY PART OF
THE REGISTER FOR FEVER NURSES.

Friday, 14th June, 1946.

MORNING PAPER.

FEVERS.

*(First Paper.)*

Time allowed 1½ hours.

**IMPORTANT.**—*Read the questions carefully, and answer only what is asked, as no marks will be given for irrelevant matter.*

*Credit will be given for simple, clear diagrams, and for legible handwriting.*

NOTE.—Three questions in all are to be answered, of which questions 1 and 2 are compulsory. Candidates who do not attempt the compulsory questions will be disqualified.

Compulsory.     1. Describe the rash of chicken-pox. How does it differ from the rash of smallpox?

Compulsory.     2. What are the main causes and varieties of puerperal infection? Give an account of the treatment of a patient suffering from sapræmia.

3. What are the common forms of influenza? How is the disease spread? Name the common complications of this disease.

4. Describe briefly the onset, course and treatment of broncho-pneumonia in a patient suffering from whooping-cough.

*Figure 3.2* Final State Examination Paper for the Supplementary Part of the Register for Fever Nurses, Friday 14 June 1946: Morning Paper, Fevers. Courtesy of Mr Alan Tobyn, son of the late Marjorie Tobyn

a nurse at Wakefield Infectious Diseases Hospital, 'sucked a tube inserted in a child's windpipe when the patient was suffering from diphtheria, in order to clear the tube and save the child from suffocation'; unfortunately, Nurse Peck then contracted the disease.[62]

It is not possible to provide accurate quantitative data of the total number of fever nurses who contracted infectious diseases; no such figures were kept

## THE GENERAL NURSING COUNCIL FOR ENGLAND AND WALES.

*The Board of Examiners by whom this paper was set is constituted as follows :—*

E. JAMES, Esq., M.D., D.P.H.                    MISS J. BLUNT, S.R.N., R.F.N.
W. GUNN, Esq., M.A., M.R.C.P., D.P.H.          MISS E. C. WHITE, S.R.N., R.F.N.

### FINAL STATE EXAMINATION FOR THE SUPPLEMENTARY PART OF THE REGISTER FOR FEVER NURSES.

*Friday, 14th June, 1946.*

AFTERNOON PAPER.
FEVER NURSING.

*(Second Paper.)*

### Time allowed 2½ hours.

**IMPORTANT.**—*Read the questions carefully, and answer only what is asked, as no marks will be given for irrelevant matter.*

*Credit will be given for simple, clear diagrams, and for legible handwriting.*

NOTE.—Five questions in all are to be answered, of which questions 1, 2 and 3 are compulsory.     Candidates who do not attempt the compulsory questions will be disqualified.

Compulsory.    1. How would you prepare for the operation of tracheotomy ? Give an account of the after-nursing.

Compulsory.    2. How would you nurse a patient suffering from scarlatinal nephritis ? At what stage of the disease is this complication likely to occur ?

Compulsory.    3. What is meant by the following :—
    (a) diaphoretic ;
    (b) hypodermic ;
    (c) infusion ;
    (d) enema ;
    (e) antitoxin.

    4. What methods may be used to reduce pyrexia ? Describe one in detail.

    5. What are the various methods of introducing drugs into the human body ? Give in detail your method of administering :—
    (a) sulphonamide tablets ;
    (b) calomel ;
    (c) magnesium sulphate.

    6. State the points which you would observe and report upon in the urine of a patient suffering from an acute febrile condition.
    How would you put up an Esbach's Albuminometer ?

*Figure 3.3* Final State Examination Paper for the Supplementary Part of the Register for Fever Nurses, Friday 14 June 1946: Afternoon Paper, Fever Nursing. Courtesy of Mr Alan Tobyn, son of the late Marjorie Tobyn

*Table 3.1* Incidence of diphtheria and scarlet fever in nursing staff, City Hospital, Edinburgh, 1919–27

| Year | Total nursing staff | Number of cases in nursing staff of | |
| | | Diphtheria | Scarlet fever |
| --- | --- | --- | --- |
| 1919 | 145 | 15 = 10.34% | 7 = 4.82% |
| 1920 | 148 | 10 = 6.75% | 14 = 9.46% |
| 1921 | 146 | 14 = 9.58% | 15 = 10.27% |
| 1922 | 147 | 13 = 8.84% | 9 = 6.12% |
| 1923 | 137 | 5 = 3.65% | 6 = 4.38% |
| 1924 | 128 | 4 = 3.12% | 11 = 8.59% |
| 1925 | 161 | 5 = 3.10% | 15 = 9.31% |
| 1926 | 153 | 2 = 1.30% | 5 = 3.26% |
| 1927 | 148 | 1 = 0.67% | 1 = 0.67% |

Source: Annual Report, Resident Physician, City Hospital, Edinburgh, 1927, p. 50

by central government departments, but many cases have been found, some of which are cited here and in other chapters. Most MOHs of small municipal hospitals, and resident medical superintendents in larger hospitals, mentioned the number of nurses affected in their annual reports, but not the rates. One exception was the City Hospital, Edinburgh, where, although standards were high, nurses still contracted diseases. In 1922–23, this hospital had 831 beds. It also had a smallpox hospital with 48 beds.[63] Table 3.1 shows that an average of 146 nurses were in employment annually in the nine-year period 1919–27, and the number and percentages of nurses affected by diphtheria and scarlet fever, the commonest infectious diseases admitted then.

The Resident Physician, Dr W. T. Benson, attributed the remarkable diminution in the incidence of scarlet fever in the nursing staff to the routine application of the diagnostic Dick test, followed by active immunisation of susceptible individuals.[64] However, he failed to include similar tables in his annual reports of 1928 and 1929, when 'six and then ten nurses went down with (mild) diphtheria!' There were also occasional, occupationally acquired, fatal illnesses among the nursing staff, including miliary TB, diphtheria, influenza and cerebro-spinal meningitis.[65] Records indicate that, well into the 1930s, the nurses were Dick tested for streptococcal resistance and were given antitoxin if necessary, and Schick tested for diphtheria; if susceptible, they then received toxoid antitoxin floccules (TAF).[66] In the eleven years up to 1934, there was a 95 per cent reduction in the number of nurses contracting diphtheria, due to active immunisation.[67]

Nationally, relatively few fever nurses appear to have succumbed to the wide range of diseases that they contracted. Those who survived may have been helped by the higher standard of care available to them. The incidence of tuberculosis began to decline in Britain after 1870, but it was still rife in some areas in the twentieth century. As some isolation hospitals had a sanatorium or special wards for tuberculous patients, nurses could contract it from their patients, or even import it into the hospital themselves. The consequence for probationers, apart from the effects of the disease, was a lengthening or discontinuation of training, either voluntarily or on medical grounds. Illness, whatever the cause, removed them from their duties, and left wards short of nursing staff. In some hospitals, it was frowned upon by the Matron and ward sisters and often regarded as a disgrace, a poor reflection of their hospital's isolation techniques. It was generally believed that the larger the hospital, the better the standard to prevent cross-infection.

## Hospital admission versus care at home

It has seldom been possible, or wise, to contain everyone with infectious diseases solely at home or in isolation hospitals. There are no data covering the whole of Britain, but in Scotland it is believed that medical and nursing care of the sick was predominantly hospital based by 1900.[68] Care at home was dependent on approval of the local MOH and the mother, or mother figure, being willing and available to provide care. In the nineteenth and early twentieth centuries, orphanhood was common because of parental death from diseases such as TB and heart disease. Women could die at, or soon after, childbirth, while accidents and suicides were more common in men. Because of this, and due to the deaths of many fathers in the First World War, a question about orphanhood was included in the census of 1921. The data revealed that, in England and Wales, the rate of persons 0–14 years orphaned by the death of one or both parents was 9.97 per cent, but in Bedfordshire, the rate was higher at 10.75 per cent.[69] Orphanhood increased the number of children requiring admission to isolation hospitals as often there was no one to care for them at home.

Confidence in hospitals was vital if the sick were not to be concealed at home and only admitted to hospital in the final stage of their illness. Such severe illness adversely affected the patient's chance of recovery and did little for the hospital's reputation. Confidence among the public appeared to be gained sooner in large city hospitals than in smaller rural institutions. In 1879, the *Lancet* stated that prejudice against hospitalisation was 'slowly but surely' wearing away. In London, resistance appeared largely to have subsided by the late 1880s. For example, it was noted in 1889 that at the MAB North Western Hospital, there was 'scarcely a vestige' of such prejudice among the socially superior classes.[70] By 1910, Miss Drakard, Matron of Plaistow Hospital, in the East End of London, a poor part of the capital, was in a position to write:

Now the people have learnt to trust the hospitals. They turn to them when their children are seriously ill, not to get rid of infection, but to obtain the best possible treatment and nursing for them. In the case of the poor this means a great deal, for, with them, the nursing of severe fever cases at home is apt to mean all-round misery. This is shown only too plainly by the state of many patients at the time they come into hospital. One cannot say they have been neglected. Indeed, the poor are nearly always very kind and self-sacrificing when there is illness in the house, but those who do the nursing have neither the means, the time, the knowledge, nor the healthy surroundings necessary for such work.[71]

In 1926, Dr Ian Thomson, the Medical Officer of Southampton Isolation Hospital, complained that a large percentage of typical cases of common infectious diseases did not arrive in hospital until three or four days after the disease had elapsed. In most cases it was a failure on the part of the parent to send for the physician until the disease was well established. He called for more education of parents.[72] The more remote the district, the greater the likelihood of late admissions into small hospitals which did not have a resident doctor, such as Biggleswade Isolation Hospital in the heart of rural Bedfordshire. In 1930, the hospital had 25 fever beds,[73] and was part of the Biggleswade Joint Hospital District, which served Biggleswade Urban and Rural (part of) and Northam Districts. A random search of hospital records reveals that the hospital was seldom full:

| | | |
|---|---|---|
| 6 August 1930 | 8 patients | (3 diphtheria, 5 scarlet fever) |
| 23 November 1932 | 10 patients | (7 scarlet fever, 3 enteric [typhoid]) |
| 14 March 1934 | no patients | |
| 29 August 1934 | 2 patients | (1 scarlet fever, 1 diphtheria) |

Most people recovered; only five patients died between July 1929 and January 1935, the period for which records survive, but they were admitted in what was described as 'a critical' or 'very critical condition' or were 'extremely ill on admission'. A boy aged 6 years (case no. 28), was admitted on 21 July 1930 with haemorrhagic diphtheria. The onset was on 18 July, when he had a sore throat and was vomiting. On admission, his throat was covered with membrane, he had a profuse nasal discharge and 'Bull neck'. Brandy 2 drachms (0.25oz) was given in the ambulance as his pulse was very poor and he was in a very serious condition. Dr Campbell, who had sent him in, had administered 8,000 units of antitoxic serum before admission. The boy's vital signs were reported, using the Fahrenheit scale, as temperature (T.) 98°F (36.6°C), pulse 128 and respirations 26 per minute. He died three days later on 24 July, with his father present. Another patient, a woman aged 41 (case no. 30), was admitted on 1 November 1932 with enteric (typhoid), found positive on bacteriological examination. No history could be given as on admission at 9 p.m., she was unconscious and dying. Observations were T. 103.6°F (39.7°C), pulse imperceptible and respirations 40. She was sent in by Dr Andrews and died at 1.45 a.m. without regaining consciousness. It was also noted that she was in a very dirty condition. Brandy was given before moving her and a hypodermic injection of Strychnine grains $\frac{1}{60}$ (1mg) was given on admission. Matron was present at the death.[74]

These two patients may have been cared for at home initially, but as their nursing and medical case notes have not survived, a complete picture is not possible. The boy (case no. 28) could have had a tracheotomy, but no mention of this has been found. The woman (case no. 30) was clearly beyond help on admission, although stimulants were given. These data, and those from Southampton, give some indication that confidence in isolation hospitals had not permeated everywhere by the 1930s.

During the 1920s, far fewer fever patients were being nursed at home, although many of the fever nurse textbooks, which had proliferated by then, still carried a section on 'Fever Nursing in Private Houses'. Although not always the case, there seems to have been an assumption by the medical authors that they were middle-class households. Dr Grace Dundas wrote in 1924 that if the nurse had a say in the choosing of the sickroom, it should have a dressing room communicating with it, both with a fireplace. The room should be of 2,000 cubic feet capacity, with large windows and a polished hard-wood floor. Details of nursing should, as far as possible, approach hospital ideals. There was a strong recommendation that the disinfectant carbolic lotion be used, in various strengths, for almost every purpose, including the patient's bedlinen, bath and the nurse's hands. The necessity to co-operate with the local sanitary authority for disinfection of the room and its contents was emphasised.[75] In 1920, two of the daughters, aged 4 and 5 years, of a Bedfordshire farmer, contracted diphtheria. Most of the family stayed at their farmhouse in Dunton, but the sisters were put into complete quarantine in their town house in Biggleswade, cared for by a nurse brought in by Dr Bridger, the local GP. As they were very ill, the doctor sat up with them all night; use was made of steam kettles and they were spared tracheotomies.[76]

One of the greatest bars in controlling the spread of infectious disease was the congregation of people together in close quarters who had not previously been subjected to such conditions. This applied especially to children at school, soldiers in barracks and nurses in hospitals. Children could be cared for in their own home, but there was no choice for those at boarding schools when the sanatorium could not cope, or soldiers and nurses who were at a distance from their home town. School attendance is known to have had a marked effect on the spread of different infectious diseases, particularly after the summer break. School registers and reports from school medical officers show that epidemics often caused schools to be closed in the latter part of the nineteenth and the first half of the twentieth centuries. Children in the early stages of an infectious disease were not always easily diagnosed. In 1930, Mabel Bedford, aged 11 years, was sent home from her junior school in Luton at lunchtime. 'I had large white spots in my throat,' she said. She was diagnosed with scarlet fever, but was frightened of going away and, as both the isolation hospitals at Luton and Dunstable were full, she was allowed to stay at home once Mr Peck, the Sanitary Inspector, had approved the arrangements. Her mother bore the brunt of the home nursing and could not go out for six weeks. She later declared, 'Never again'.[77]

The outbreak of the First World War in August 1914 meant that soldiers were mobilised from rural areas, where infection was more easily contained, to urban areas. Not only were they living in close proximity to each other, but also through mixing with townspeople, they were easy prey to childhood infections. Fever hospitals were soon full of sick soldiers, so other hospitals had to be converted to provide care for them. For example the Territorial Highland Division moved from small Scottish communities to Bedford, which had a large juvenile population. Hundreds of soldiers contracted a virulent form of measles and 85 men died between the beginning of the autumn term and the end of November 1914. Valuable assistance was given by members of a local Voluntary Aid Detachment (VAD), who acted as unpaid orderlies, freeing the nurses to carry out patient care.[78] In Luton, there was a serious outbreak of diphtheria. In order to prevent the troops, who were billeted in private houses and camps, entering infected houses, large red crosses were painted on the doors. Gertrude Simmons (born 1904) contracted the disease. Her mother wrung a cloth out in carbolic and hung it at her bedroom door, but her two brothers contracted the disease, 'their curiosity being too much for the flimsy barrier'.[79] Most mothers, because they had to remain isolated with their children were not keen to repeat the experience.

A similar situation emerged in the Second World War. For example, epidemics affected soldiers from the town barracks in Dunstable and boys from Dunstable Grammar School, who were boarders. Such patients were rarely homesick; once they began to recover they were quite happy.[80] The first wave of West Indian nurses came to Bedfordshire in the mid-1950s to undergo general nurse training at Luton and Dunstable Hospital, where they were required to be resident in the nurses' home. When they were seconded to the Children's Annexe, some contracted infectious diseases and were sent to Spittlesea Isolation Hospital, and afterwards to convalesce at Edgebury Hospital, near Woburn Sands.[81] A number of examples have been given of the very variable care available, either at home or in hospital. Children were often nursed at home, sometimes because conditions were declared suitable by the local MOH, but more often because an epidemic meant that there were insufficient hospital beds, even when tents were used.

Comparative mortality rates are the main indicators of effective care, although other mitigating factors, such as the admission of patients in a dying state, are seldom mentioned. In the decennial period 1906–15, in Mirfield, West Yorkshire, there were 623 notifications of scarlet fever. Of these, 94 per cent were treated in hospital and 6 per cent at home. The death rate of all cases was 2.4 per cent, but only 1.4 percent for those treated in hospital.[82] In 1936, the new MOH for Luton, Fred Grundy, prepared a very comprehensive annual report with a table purportedly giving data concerning diphtheria notifications for the decennial period, 1927–36, but which included other significant information. According to Grundy, it was not unlikely that 'the recent great growth in the population of Luton has affected

*Table 3.2* Diphtheria notifications in Luton and death rates in Luton and in England and Wales, 1927–36

|  | 1927 | 1928 | 1929 | 1930 | 1931 | 1932 | 1933 | 1934 | 1935 | 1936 |
|---|---|---|---|---|---|---|---|---|---|---|
| Notified | 190 | 210 | 99 | 147 | 68 | 26 | 105 | 415 | 283 | 400 |
| Attack rate | 3.22 | 3.29 | 1.50 | 2.25 | 0.98 | 0.37 | 1.47 | 5.45 | 3.53 | 4.67 |
| Admitted to hospital | 125 | 128 | 64 | 104 | 50 | 18 | 89 | 334 | 248 | 386 |
| Nursed at home | 65 | 82 | 35 | 43 | 18 | 8 | 16 | 81 | 35 | 14 |
| Number of deaths | 9 | 11 | 3 | 6 | 4 | 2 | 8 | 32 | 16 | 39 |
| Death rate | 0.18 | 0.18 | 0.06 | 0.09 | 0.05 | 0.02 | 0.11 | 0.42 | 0.19 | 0.45 |
| Death rate (England and Wales) | 0.07 | 0.06 | 0.08 | 0.09 | 0.07 | 0.06 | 0.06 | 0.10 | 0.08 | 0.07 |

Source: Annual Report, Medical Officer of Health, Borough of Luton, 1936, Table III Particulars of diphtheria notifications since 1927, p. 90

the mass immunity of what was relatively a closed community'. This could account for the increased incidence and severity of the disease (see Table 3.2).

These data not only show an increased incidence of diphtheria after 1932, but also reveal a higher death rate in the borough than in England and Wales from 1933, probably due to the influx of workers to the town from the depressed areas seeking work. Table 3.2 also shows that 1,546 children were nursed in the local hospital, but 397 (26 per cent) were cared for at home. The 39 deaths in 1936, apparently due to a severe form of the disease, 'Diphtheria Gravis', were not attributed to home or hospital.[83] Patients' views about their locus of care were seldom considered.

## Patients' perspectives

The recent use of oral evidence from patients in nursing history provides valuable additional sources of information and a different perspective, but these are dependent on time to collect them before it is too late and, as with all oral testimony, the vagaries of the human memory. By the twentieth century, more former patients who had recovered from infectious diseases were ready to publish or otherwise share their experiences, often on reflection, many years later. This particular genre has seldom been properly explored in nursing as a tool to further understanding of the past and, even here, only a few examples can be given.

In 1982, a 68-year-old woman recalled the nine weeks that she spent in hospital in 1918 with scarlet fever at the age of 4½ years, but there is no indication in the article as to which hospital or its location. Nevertheless, her experiences may be fairly typical of care then. Collected by a fever van, her first experience of being out in the dark and in a motor vehicle, but not a word of kindness or explanation was spoken to her by the nurse, or to the little boy who was also picked up and laid on the other shelf. At the hospital, the two children were both undressed, immersed in cloudy disinfectant water, too hot to bear, and given a good scrub with a large brush. The girl had her long hair cut short before it was 'dunked' into the water. Admitted into adjacent beds, she wailed for her mother, while screens were placed around his bed. The next morning, the boy in the bed on the other side of her told her that the little boy had died in the night. She imagined that that was to be her fate. A further series of unpleasant events in hospital, including the lack of visitors at the bedside and being smacked repeatedly, resulted in her losing her speech. Because she was so frightened, the only word she uttered during this long hospital stay was 'Mother'. She is convinced that 'the terrors experienced as a four-year-old child' had lifelong physical and psychological effects.[84]

Another former patient, writing in 1984 at the age of 76 years, commented about her experience with diphtheria at the local fever hospital at Otford in Kent, in 1919, when she was 11 years old. She particularly remembers the doctor not being called for five days after she became ill because of the cost of a home visit – seven shillings and sixpence (37.5p) – and being collected by the dreaded 'fever cart' from her home after dark. Her father owned a butcher's shop and 'feared that he would be ruined as nobody would buy their meat from a shop where there might be diphtheria germs lurking'. She felt that the Isolation Hospital for Sevenoaks Rural Area, in Kent, was very primitive. It still used a horse-drawn ambulance and did not have a telephone, which made communication between the doctor and the hospital, and the hospital and parents, very difficult. It was a very small establishment with one three-bedded and one five-bedded ward for scarlet fever and an identical building for patients with diphtheria. There were also 'little galvanised iron huts', each with one bed for isolation of typhoid, smallpox or other unusual complaints. This girl was the only patient at first, but later two little girls and one boy were admitted, all seriously ill. When one girl died the gardener had to walk to her house to inform her parents. Her five weeks' stay does not appear to have been as traumatic as that experienced by the previous patient, apart from the shock she had when she was unable to return home with her own books and toys, especially her teddy bear. This hospital, which had nineteen beds, apparently provided work for the Matron, two nurses, two maids, laundry staff and a gardener.[85]

In 1929, Elizabeth, then aged 14 years, was admitted to Spittlesea Isolation Hospital in Luton, where she was ill for some weeks with scarlet fever. Ten days after she returned home she developed diphtheria, which her 19-year-old brother George contracted. Elizabeth and her brother were admitted as they, and their four other siblings, were orphans and there was no one to care for them at home. He was in hospital for four weeks, during which time a 2-year-old child choked to death in his six-bedded ward. He has never forgotten this incident and even at 93 years of age, he still refers to it.[86]

Admission to an isolation hospital was often a devastating experience; generally, the younger the child, the greater the traumatic effect. In common with other types of hospital for the physically ill, until after the Second World War, priority was usually given to bodily requirements, not psychological or emotional needs.

## Pay and conditions of service

Improvements in pay and conditions of service came about largely to increase the number, and improve the calibre, of nursing staff in both large and small isolation hospitals. Throughout its history, 1867–1930, the MAB in London was never free from the major problem of staffing the wards.[87] The better the residential accommodation, with amenities such as central heating and bathrooms, the more likely it was that a young woman from a higher social class than domestic servants, from which nurses were previously drawn, would be attracted. Moreover, by the early twentieth century a fever nurse could have more than elementary schooling: the Education Act, 1902, gave working-class children in England and Wales the opportunity of a grammar school education. Young women were more likely to apply to train at a large isolation hospital with up-to-date facilities, which had a similar, but somewhat inferior, social cachet to the large voluntary hospital. Young nurses who worked in small hospitals were disadvantaged in different ways; there were usually fewer resources, and some endured dormitory-like accommodation or cubicles. However, most nurses in all branches of the profession were required to live in nurses' homes until the 1960s and often beyond.

Salary scales seemed low at times, as the residential accommodation with all meals provided was not always taken into account. Nevertheless, salaries were often somewhat higher in fever hospitals than in other institutions. In the absence of national scales, hospitals paid the minimum rate necessary to secure and retain staff. During a smallpox epidemic in London in 1869–70, the MAB decided to erect a temporary hospital in Hampstead with 90 beds – extendable to 180 beds if necessary. The hospital opened in January 1870, with nuns taking on the nursing and domestic work. Their rate of pay at the new Hampstead Smallpox Hospital was higher than that at the London Fever Hospital, which was filled to capacity, and where many of the staff had contracted the disease. The MAB was criticised by the Poor Law Board for its liberality, but reminded the Board that 'the engagements are entirely of a temporary character ... and the employment is not without considerable personal risk'.[88] Table 3.3 shows that the MAB continued to pay higher salaries in comparison to some other large fever hospitals in Britain in the 1890s.

The variable annual rates payable to probationers were, it seems, governed by the law of supply and demand. In 1913, the FNA provided all the Fever Hospital Committees in the United Kingdom with recommendations for minimum salaries to be paid to nurses in fever hospitals. Probationers

*Table 3.3* Annual salaries (£) for probationers in some large British fever
hospitals, 1890s

|  | 1st year | 2nd year | 3rd year |
| --- | --- | --- | --- |
| Cork Street Fever Hospital, Dublin – 1895 | 12 | 15 | — |
| City Hospital, Edinburgh – 1899 | 16 | 19 | 22 |
| Glasgow Fever and Smallpox Hospitals – 1899 | 18 | 24 | — |
| MAB fever hospitals - 1899 (Class II assistant nurses)* | 24 | 25 | — |

Source: National Library of Ireland, Dublin, 'The Nurses of the Irish Hospitals: No. VIII –
Nursing School of Cork Street Fever Hospital', *The Lady of the House*, 15 June 1895, p. 3, and
*Burdett's Hospitals and Charities, 1899*
Note: *The MAB had not begun training its own probationers in 1899; Class II assistant
nurses were the nearest equivalent

should receive £18 in the first year and £20 in the second, plus indoor
uniform.[89] Appendix 3 provides further evidence of the lack of standard rates
of pay for fever nurses in hospitals in England and Wales in August 1919. Of
the ten hospitals cited, which ranged from 30 to 623 beds, four were managed
by the MAB, which paid the highest salary, although uniform was not
provided. Salaries for first-year probationers ranged from £20 to £40 per
annum. Monsall Fever Hospital (365 beds), Manchester, paid the lowest
rate, although it did provide indoor uniform. Direct comparisons between
hospitals are, therefore, difficult to make due to the difference in uniform
provision, seen then as a benefit, not a right. However, overall the salaries of
fever nurses were improved by the efforts of the FNA in the years leading up
to state registration.[90]

In 1930, the average pay of fever nurse probationers in hospitals approved
for training was £32 1s 0d (£32.05) in the first year and £37 12s 0d (£37.60)
in the second year, a much higher rate than probationers in hospitals
approved for special children's training and voluntary hospitals in London
and in the provinces. This could be taken as a form of weighting due to the
health risks involved. Probationers in approved municipal and tuberculosis
hospitals received almost as much as those in fever training.[91] It is clear that
when recruitment was a particular problem, as it was in the 1930s, salaries
were improved. As was seen earlier, the TUC wanted to secure a forty-eight-
hour week for nurses, but the RCN opposed the initiative.

During the Second World War, a committee was set up in 1943 under Lord
Rushcliffe (with a similar committee in Scotland under Professor Taylor) to
consider the salaries of trained nurses and those in training; it also examined
conditions of service and salaries for assistant nurses and auxiliaries. The
Report of the Nurses Salaries Committee 1943 'became the starting point for
negotiations, and for the first Nurses and Midwives Whitley Council in 1948'.
The Rushcliffe Committee recommended improved salary scales for all
grades and proposed that the working fortnight be reduced to ninety-six
hours, that continuous night duty should not exceed six months for trained

staff and three months for student nurses. Every nurse should be entitled to twenty-eight days' annual leave with one day off duty every week and sick pay graded according to length of service. Higher grade salaries were to be paid according to the number of beds, a principle followed for the next 30 years.[92]

The recommendations made in the Report of the Nurses Salaries Committee, 1943, may have been difficult to implement in some small isolation hospitals, but a number of large city hospitals in Britain had already introduced, or exceeded, some of these measures. By 1926–27, general conditions offered by the MAB included four weeks' annual leave and two days off duty per week. Practically all nurses were promised a separate bedroom or cubicle and the amenities included 'conference, dining, lecture and recreation rooms, together with facilities for outdoor games'. Salaries for probationers were £29 and £31 respectively, in the first and second years of training; sisters were paid a salary ranging from £80 to £95 and staff nurses £60–70 per annum with an additional £5 for their specialist fever nurse qualification and extra pay when nursing smallpox patients. Registered and assistant nurses were entitled to extra payments of £2 per annum after five years' service and an additional £10 annually after ten years' service. Other benefits included the return of board money when on leave, guaranteed ample sickness benefits ('better than the state scheme') and the opportunity to join a pension scheme.[93]

## Effect of the National Health Service, 1948

The National Health Service Act, 1946, was not implemented until 'the appointed day', 5 July 1948. Management of municipal isolation hospitals and smallpox hospitals was then transferred from local authorities to joint hospital management committees, under the control of regional hospital boards. Charles Webster, a health care historian, observed that 'the National Health Service profoundly reduced the part played by local authorities in health care'. He believed that this was traumatic for them, as it represented a sudden and unexpected reversal of policies which had been followed since the early twentieth century. The largest losses experienced by local authorities were in Poor Law, general, tuberculosis, infectious diseases, mental and mental deficiency hospitals and institutions.[94] Nevertheless, it could be argued that the NHS provided a catalyst for necessary change in fever nursing. There was increasing recognition that isolation measures in separate hospitals were seldom required; these could be provided in a general hospital with readier access to other services such as X-ray and pathology. Rationalisation would leave fewer, but more specialised isolation hospitals. Many small isolation hospitals were, therefore, closed, while others were used for different purposes, for example, convalescent or geriatric patients. Nurses with general and fever nurse qualifications were more likely to find employment, perhaps, in infection control, than those with only the RFN certificate.

## Closure of fever registers

The Nursing Reconstruction Committee, set up in 1941 by the RCN under the chairmanship of Lord Horder, had two fever nurses on the Kindred Associations Panel of Representatives, Miss E. Barcham, League of Fever Nurses, and Miss A. Ward, Infectious Hospitals Matrons' Association (IHMA). They were involved in the recommendation to enrol assistant nurses under the control of the GNC for England and Wales, which resulted in the Nurses Act, 1943,[95] and which later caused single qualified RFNs such concern as it also involved a two-year course. In fact, the League of Fever Nurses had sent a letter protesting against the enrolment of semi-trained assistant nurses and their recognition by the state. The League was described (probably by Mrs Fenwick) in an editorial footnote as, 'This group of highly efficient Fever Nurses [who] were never consulted by the Minister of Health . . . so detrimental to their interests and to those of their patients'.[96] The Horder Report (1943) also recommended a four-year training for general nurses with 'experience in obstetric nursing and such branches as mental, fever and tuberculosis nursing with an elective six months in a speciality during the final year'. It was envisaged that once this wider type of training was available, other parts of the register should be closed.[97]

By 1948, it was a foregone conclusion that fever nurse training would soon cease. In fact, the first meeting to discuss the closure of the Fever Register in England and Wales had already taken place between representatives of the GNC and the Ministry of Health on 24 November 1947, but closure was not effected until 31 December 1967. In the interim period, student nurses continued to be taken on courses approved by the GNC, despite growing evidence that the future of this specialism was uncertain. There had been an enormous decline in most common infectious diseases, partly as a result of more effective immunisation campaigns and the introduction of antibiotics. More importantly, partly as a result of wartime food rationing, better nutrition resulted in better health; many people were, therefore, more likely to resist infection, or if affected, not to succumb as readily. Improved living conditions meant that more children were able to be nursed at home. Nevertheless, the seriously ill still needed specialist care. Certainly, the postwar epidemics of poliomyelitis prolonged the life of some isolation hospitals.

The various factions concerned with the projected closure of the Fever Nurses' Register expressed considerable anxiety. The first issue focused on the maintenance of skilled infectious nursing once the register was closed, a particular concern of the IHMA and the British College of Nurses (BCN). There was a consensus view that fever nurse training should be part of the general nurse course by rotation. By 1952, Oxford Regional Hospital Board had already implemented such a scheme. The second issue was concerned with the maintenance of a labour force. Some management committees were known to be particularly concerned with staffing hospitals with 'sufficient pairs of hands hitherto provided by student nurses'. The Resident Physician of Ham Green Hospital, near Bristol, observed that without nurses seconded from Bristol Royal Infirmary, they could never have kept their wards open.[98]

An experimental scheme for training fever nurses at Joyce Green Hospital, Dartford, previously an infectious diseases hospital with 1,104 beds, was approved by the Ministry of Health and the GNC in April 1952. As this hospital already had a unit for treating patients with infectious diseases, nurses in general training could acquire three months' experience in fevers which, with an extra nine months' post-general registration training, would result in two certificates, those of the state registered nurse (SRN) and RFN. Students could, therefore, shorten their period of specialist training,[99] an inducement for them, but from a management perspective, the strategy ensured retention of staff for a longer period.

In 1953, concern grew in the IHMA about the likely closure of the register. In July, Ada Ward, the president, sent a letter about the situation to all members. In reply to a letter and Resolution of Protest against the proposed closure of the Fever Nurses' Register, sent by the association to the Minister of Health and important medical associations, encouraging responses had been received promising help and support. Nevertheless, it was deemed sufficiently important to unify all interested parties, and fully qualified fever nurses were now to be included in the renamed body, the Infectious Hospitals Matrons' and Nurses' Association (IHMNA). New members, such as sisters and staff nurses, were now welcome to 'help in revising the importance of adequate recognition of this splendid branch of our Profession'.[100] New by-laws were issued which included the aim 'to take action if necessary upon legislative proposals which affect the interests of Nurses in the Infectious Hospitals'.[101]

Despite knowing that the closure of the Fever Nurse Register was imminent, the GNC for England and Wales still issued a new syllabus in 1954. For the first time, the GNC acknowledged the fact known by most fever nurses, that 'the majority of patients in infectious diseases hospitals are children'. The syllabus introduced a minimum of 4 hours' lectures in paediatrics, to be given by a registered medical practitioner (if possible one holding a Diploma in Child Health), a small part of the total 54 class hours required. The topics listed in the syllabus included development of the normal child, variations from the normal, observation and handling of infants and children, and feeding of infants and children in health and disease. Lecturers were also referred to the dietetics part of the syllabus.[102] In spite of joint schemes of training and amendments to the syllabus, a series of statistics pointed to the inevitability of the closure of the Fever Nurse Register in England and Wales.

In the year ending 1960, the average duration of stay in infectious disease hospitals in England and Wales was only 18.6 days; there were 7,266 staffed beds, but only 3,458 were in use. Inquiries made into 23 hospitals approved for fever nurse training showed that on 15 February 1962, only 1,538 beds were occupied by patients suffering from infectious diseases (excluding tuberculosis). Moreover, only 180 cases fell into the group of specific fevers most common in infectious disease hospitals in the early twentieth century: scarlet fever, diphtheria, measles, chickenpox, whooping cough and mumps. The remainder of the infectious disease cases included 54 patients with poliomyelitis, 445 with a wide assortment of gastro-intestinal infections, plus many with pneumonia and upper respiratory tract infections. Of the other 1,919 patients, 504 had chest diseases, including tuberculosis, and 1,415 were classified as ear, nose and throat patients or geriatrics. Moreover, the number of students entering for the final examinations for fever nursing had declined from 227 in 1955–56 to 177 in 1960–61.[103]

For various reasons, some nurses who had completed approved fever nurse courses failed to register; some had not reached 21 years, the age at which they could register, and others assumed that registration was automatic. Sometimes it was only the Matron of the hospital they had entered for general training who informed them that registration was necessary before a one-year remission could be allowed. It was not unusual to have a gap between qualification and registration. For example, fever nurse number 21,505 trained at Moxley Hospital, Wednesbury, between 1956 and 1958, but did not register until 31 December 1967, the date on which the Fever Register for England and Wales was closed.[104]

It is clear from analysis of the Fever Nurse Registers for England and Wales in London, and for Scotland in Edinburgh, that there was obvious haste to record qualifications before it was too late. The Scottish Fever Nurse Register closed one year after that of England and Wales. The last nurse to be entered on 31 December 1968 (E28,708) qualified at Groby Hospital, Leicester, between 1962 and 1964. The last nurse to register (E28,704) who qualified in Scotland in 1953 trained at the County Hospital, Invergordon.[105] There had been a similar but slightly later decline in training in the Irish Republic, where the Supplementary Register for Fever Nurses, 'Infectious Diseases Division', was closed in 1971.[106]

In Northern Ireland, there was some concern that closure of the register might lower the standard of fever nursing, for which there was still some demand, but it was realised that there was a very limited potential for employment in this speciality in the United Kingdom. As it was impractical to continue, the decision was made to close the register in January 1970; this was confirmed by Statutory Order in 1972 and the last name was entered in 1973.[107]

In the Irish Republic, some additional names were added to the Register of Nurses in Infectious Disease, up to and including 1976, the final year it was maintained. Some of those listed trained in Great Britain and Northern Ireland. Of the total number of 1,809 names entered on this register between 1921 and 1976, all were female.[108] The variation in length of training indicated that it was either carried out as a post-basic course (one year) or as an initial course (two years). All the fever nurse registers in the United Kingdom and in the Irish Republic are now closed, but some nurses are still able to make good use of their qualification. Although sounding distinctly outmoded, the term 'fever nurse' survives. Data published annually by the Nursing and Midwifery Council, the regulatory professional body for Nursing, Midwifery and Health Visiting in the United Kingdom (it does not cover the Irish Republic) still includes the Professional Register, Part 9, 'Fever nurses'. As of 31 March 2003, there were still 107 nurses with this single qualification and 529 entered in fever nursing and another, unspecified, part of the register. The overwhelming predominance of females in this branch of nursing may be seen in a gender analysis of these 529 nurses, of whom 523 (99 per cent) were female with only 6 (1 per cent) male.[109]

## Conclusion

This chapter has covered a period of great change in society, including two world wars, Irish devolution, the emancipation of women, the introduction of antibiotics and the inception of the NHS. The passage of Bills for state registration came to fruition in 1919, eighteen years after the Nurses Registration Act, 1901, in New Zealand. Some schisms which already existed in the nursing profession in Britain before registration, were perpetuated by the differences in the duration of fever nurse training in Scotland (three years) and the two years thought necessary in other parts of Britain, as Scottish matrons were protective of their own schemes. For the most part, doctors were a source of helpful professional advice for fever nurses, and for the advancement of fever nursing. Nevertheless, tremendous underlying tension can be sensed in official reports in the period 1921–24, not least because some medical men, representing the Society of MOHs in Scotland, reneged on their intention to support Scottish matrons.

Once the issue was resolved, reciprocity became possible between Scotland and other countries in the British Isles, and internationally, where state-approved schemes existed in general nursing with fever experience. Scotland and Ireland were successful in their bids to retain autonomy and not to be subject to control from London, hence the three separate GNCs. Although the GNCs made provision for combined (or integrated) courses, there was relatively little uptake; most fever nurses undertook the basic two-year scheme, although some opted for the one-year course following general training.

The LGB recommendation of one isolation bed per thousand persons in 1882 resulted in almost insuperable dilemmas, particularly for small local authorities expected to staff isolation hospitals. This led to the virtual necessity for two different kinds of fever nurse training. Large hospitals were able to gain approval from their relevant professional body, unlike small hospitals, whose resources were insufficient to support an approved scheme. Large hospitals needed far more probationers, but were more likely to attract them because of a properly validated course which could reduce the length of another course, particularly general nurse training, and because they usually had better residential accommodation and other amenities. As was seen in Table 3.3 and in Appendix 3, the MAB could offer higher salaries. The Board dominated the FNA, but derived from it the wisdom to manage its own courses. It proved to be a model employer of fever nurses. However, its control as a training authority was greatly diluted when its powers were assumed by the GNC. Nevertheless, the MAB, and after 1930, the London County Council (LCC), continued to conduct their own hospital examinations and issue certificates (see Appendix 4.3 and 4.6), in much the same way as other fever hospitals in Britain and the Irish Republic.

National bodies in Scotland and Ireland, which had previously validated fever nurse courses, and the FNA, an independent association, and their successors, the GNCs, influenced by powerful matrons of large hospitals, metaphorically 'washed their hands' of the training needs of small hospitals. However, much to the chagrin of the GNC for England and Wales, the Ministry of Health showed that it, really, held the power by overruling decisions it had made regarding approval for training at Darlington and Hastings, an anomalous situation considering that Scotland had campaigned for a three-year course.

To a large extent, men were excluded from fever nursing; this would seem to lend support to Abel-Smith's 1960 thesis that when women attained power they used it to discriminate against men. However, one of the effects of the Second World War was a change in attitudes to previously held social norms. Men began to enter fever nursing, not as *ab initio* apprentices, but often with valuable experience as medical orderlies. They could have brought new ideas and treatments with them to benefit fever nursing, but it is unlikely that these would have been welcomed from them in their subservient role. Almost certainly, their presence alone caused consternation at times.

The strategy of training nurses to maintain the workforce has been deprecated, but there was little option for employers; fever nurse probationers were, in reality, 'pairs of hands', more than students, although they were termed that since the 1940s. The ethics of some managers and matrons must be questioned. They often appeared to have 'forgotten' to inform candidates that training that was not approved by the GNC would prevent them from being eligible for a shortened general training. Moreover, between 1947 and the closure of the fever registers, there seems to have been collusion to keep both male and female candidates in ignorance about the likely end of fever nurse training to ensure that hospitals remained open. The other issue which disadvantaged fever nurses was the age at which they could register. In 1920, the GNC for England and Wales decided that the minimum age for state registration, for all branches of nursing, should be 21 years. As the age for the two-year fever training course was lowered to 17 years in the 1930s, it led to the situation where some nurses registered very late or not at all. There are no national data of fever nurses who did not complete courses. The reasons are varied, as will be seen in Chapter 4.

The health risks borne by fever nurses at work cannot be laid solely at the door of isolation hospitals; although infectious diseases were present there, they were often rife in the communities where they took their off duty and annual leave. Nevertheless, the likelihood of sickness was a factor of which they were unlikely to have been warned at selection interview, as recruitment was usually difficult. Morbidity and mortality figures concerning isolation hospital staff, had they existed centrally and been published, might have considerably hampered recruitment initiatives. Fever hospitals used the same strategies as other institutions to attract labour in the form of probationers: improved living conditions, better conditions of service and contracts for training (the most successful ploy). However, pay in many isolation hospitals exceeded that in other hospitals, including what was really 'danger money' for those who, heroically, nursed smallpox patients. Only the nurses involved could say if the end (contracting an infectious disease) justified the means.

The issues of concealment of seriously ill people at home, and late admission leading to early death, delayed confidence in isolation hospitals, but it is not possible from the few cases cited here to decide whether care at home or in hospital was more effective. Again, the lack of quantitative data prevents statistically accurate conclusions from being drawn. Although only a few patients' experiences are cited here, they highlight the harsh impact of sudden admission, poorly understood hospital practices and deaths of neighbouring patients on those unused to hospital life, and underline the adverse effect on patients. Many fever nurses were undoubtedly kind and understanding, but some lacked empathy; the psychological needs of patients were seldom found in the curriculum until the 1950s.

Once the autonomy of local authorities was lost in 1948, isolation and smallpox hospitals began to be closed. Decisions were taken without much consultation with nurses. Despite representations from professional fever nurse bodies, the fever registers were closed. Society had changed to a large extent. Ostensibly, the general public was healthier, with better immunity, improved housing, access to a free health care service and reliance on the new antibiotics. Fever nursing in separate hospitals was not considered necessary; the wisdom of this is now questioned. Throughout their existence, isolation hospitals put patients at risk of contracting a more serious, perhaps life-threatening disease, than the one for which they were admitted. It remained to be seen if this problem would be any better once patients were transferred to other institutions. However, it is important to emphasise that fever nurses made a positive contribution to the nation's health which, together with advances in medical science, prevented many physical complications and some deaths, and enabled patients to live worthwhile lives.

## Notes and references*

1 Susan Villiers' address as president of the Fever Nurses' Association at the annual meeting, held on 23 May 1925, *British Journal of Nursing*, June 1925: 124.
2 Baly (1995), p. 145.
3 Baly (1980), pp. 153–54. The BNA became the Royal British Nurses' Association (RBNA) in 1893.
4 Ibid., pp. 154–55.
5 Donahue (1996), pp. 294–95, and information from Dr Pamela Wood, Associate Professor, Graduate School of Nursing and Midwifery, Victoria University of Wellington, New Zealand.
6 Maclean (1932). This book is the seminal text on state registration in New Zealand.
7 Schorr and Kennedy (1999), pp. 17–18, and information from Dr Brigid Lusk, Associate Professor, Northern Illinois University, Illinois.
8 J. Lynaugh, 'Fever Hospitals and Fever Nurses in Britain' (personal communication by email,17 March 2004). Joan Lynaugh, RN, PhD, FAAN, is Emeritus Professor and Associate Director, Center for the Study of the History of Nursing, University of Pennsylvania, Philadelphia, PA.
9 McGann (1992), p. 26.
10 Ibid., pp. 43–44.
11 C. Maggs (1981) 'The Register of Nurses in the Scottish Poor Law Service 1885–1919', *Nursing Times*, 25 November: 129–32.
12 The Act of Union with England and Wales and Scotland took place in 1707; the Act of Union with Ireland followed in 1800, thus establishing the United Kingdom of Great Britain and Ireland.
13 Cook and Stevenson (1988), pp. 256–59, 314.
14 *BJN*, 24 June 1916: 550. This information, drawn from the annual report of the FNA, 1915–16, contains much more detail about these issues.
15 McGann (1992), pp. 2, 27.
16 Gray (1999), p. 354.
17 See, for example, *BJN*, 24 June, 1916: 551–52.
18 Scanlan (1991), pp. 88–90.
19 McGann (1992), p. 151.
20 The Midwives (Ireland) Act, 1918, had already provided for the regulation of midwifery training and practice through the establishment of a Central Midwives Board for Ireland.
21 The name 'Eire' was used from 1922, when independence was attained, until 1937, the year when (Southern) Ireland declared itself a Republic, but the term 'Eire' tended to be used internationally, even after 1937. The Irish Free State was an alternative term used until 1937. It is now properly termed the Republic of Ireland or the Irish Republic.
22 Bendall and Raybould (1969), p. 38.
23 Abel-Smith (1960), p. 114.
24 Dingwall et al. (1988), p. 90, and discussed further in Rafferty (1996).
25 Dingwall et al. (1988), p. 91.
26 Gray (1999), pp. 143, 156, 354.

*———
Full references appear in the Bibliography.

27 Edinburgh University Library, LHSC MAC/GD 1/46/1–3; GD 1/26/2/4, and LHB 1/97/5. Miss Samuel went on to complete a three-year general nursing course at the Royal Infirmary, Edinburgh (1922–25), reduced from the usual Scottish norm of a four-year period due to her previous fever nurse training.

28 KCLA/RBNA/2/2 AGM Minutes, June 1917 – June 1947. RBNA Annual Report, 1921.

29 Scottish Record Office (SRO), Edinburgh General Nursing Council (GNC) 3/1 Annual Report, GNC for Scotland to the Scottish Board of Health, 1921.

30 SRO, GNC 3/1 Annual Report GNC for Scotland, 1922.

31 National Archives/Public Record Office NA/PRO/DT5/232, Part 2, GNC for England and Wales, Education and Examinations Committee Minutes, p. 351: Meeting, 27 February 1923.

32 SRO, GNC 3/1 Annual Report GNC for Scotland, 1923.

33 *Nursing Times and Journal of Midwifery*, 21 May 1924: pp. 489–90.

34 SRO, GNC 3/1 Annual Report GNC for Scotland, 1924.

35 SRO, GNC 3/1 Annual Report GNC for Scotland, 1925.

36 Archives of An Bord Altranais, Dublin. MS GNC for Ireland. Register of Nurses for the sick formed and kept under the provision of the Nurses Act, 1950, Supplementary Part Containing the Names of Nurses trained in the Nursing of persons suffering from Infectious Diseases.

37 Training at the Pennsylvania Fever Hospital was part of a four-year training undertaken at the Belfriar Union Infirmary. The register indicates that the candidate nurses (who were small in number) entered on to the Supplementary Register for Nurses trained in the Nursing of persons suffering from Infectious Diseases, obtained six months' fever training at the Belfriar Union and six months at the Pennsylvania Fever Hospital. This was clearly a combined training. It also shows that there were still a number of patients at the Belfriar Union with infectious diseases, despite having a separate fever hospital in the city.

38 Robins (2000), p. 20.

39 I am greatly indebted to Dr Gerard Fealy, the Irish nurse historian, of University College Dublin, who examined the records concerning fever nurses at the Archives of An Bord Altranais, Dublin in 2003 on my behalf, with the assistance of Mr Vincent Breheny, an Education Officer at the Board.

40 See for example Appendix 4.10, the certificate of a nurse at Dublin Fever Hospital, 1957–59; the two-year programme clearly continued.

41 In the early 1950s, Cork Street Fever Hospital, Dublin, was relocated to a new site in West County Dublin and was variously referred to as the Dublin Fever Hospital, Clondalkin, Ballyfermot, the Dublin Fever Hospital, Cherry Orchard or simply, Cherry Orchard Hospital. Data regarding training from nurse, 5 January 1997.

42 Dublin Health Authority. Cherry Orchard Hospital, Ballyfermot, Dublin. Hospital certificate, Miss Margaret Waters, 3 October 1962 to 3 October 1964, and her transcript of training.

43 Bendall and Raybould (1969), pp. 39, 87. *Burdett's Hospitals and Charities, 1929*, gives 1926 as the date of discontinuation of FNA examinations, but a more accurate source is the *BJN*, June 1925: 125, which cites it as 1925.

44 Maggs, op. cit., p. 132.

45 *BJN*, June 1925: 124–25. A reference to unqualified nurses who had gained experience in the First World War in a Voluntary Aid Detachment and who, trained nurses feared, would apply for state registration and thus usurp their role.

46 Ibid.

47 NA/PRO MH55/467. 93261/3/47, Darlington Infectious Diseases Hospital. Refusal of GNC to approve as a training centre. Appeal under Section 7(2) of the Nurses Registration Act, 1919: 1925–26.

48 NA/PRO MH55/468. 93261/3/48, Hastings Infectious Diseases Hospital: refusal of GNC to approve as a training centre. Appeal under Section 7(2) of the Nurses Registration Act, 1919.

49 Ibid.

50 *The Hospitals Year-Book, 1935*, pp. 278–80.

51 Ayers (1971), p. 147.

52 Abel-Smith (1960), pp. 114, 117, ref. 3. Abel-Smith is a highly regarded historian of the nursing profession.

53 Baly (1995), p. 206. Baly gives the closure of the Register for Fever Nurses in England and Wales as 1966; it was 31 December 1967.

54 Abel-Smith (1960), p. 143.

55 Syllabus of Lectures and Demonstrations for Education and Training in Fever Nursing. GNC for England and Wales, London, 1923.

56 Syllabus of Subjects for Examination for the Certificate of Fever Nursing. GNC for England and Wales, London, 1954.

57 NA/PRO DT10/176 Register of Fever Nurses no. 4. This male nurse, no. 17,472, came from Essex. He, and the other three male fever nurses whose names were recorded in 1948, all trained at the County Sanatorium and Isolation Hospital, Markfield, Leicester.

58 NA/PRO MH55/2114. Memo dated 14 June 1949.

59 Search carried out at An Bord Altranais by Dr Gerard Fealy, University College Dublin.

60 Annual Report, County MOH, Bedfordshire, 1900, p. 31. George Newman became Chief Medical Officer of the Board of Education 1907–35 and additionally, Chief Medical Officer of the Ministry of Health 1919–35.

61 *BJN*, 9 May 1914: 408. After 1902, gloves were used there in the scarlet fever and diphtheria wards for all throat treatments and for dressings. See Porter (1997), p. 373, for a short discussion on the early use of rubber gloves in surgery in North America and in Britain.

62 *Wakefield Express* and *West Riding Herald*, July 1910, mentioned in a lecture to the History of Nursing Group at the RCN, London, in May 1985 by D. J. Westmancoat, Information Officer, British Library Newspaper Library, *The History of Nursing Group at the Royal College of Nursing, Bulletin 8*, autumn 1985, p. 6.

63 *Burdett's Hospitals and Charities, 1922–23*.

64 Annual Report of the Medical Superintendent, City Hospital, Edinburgh, 1927, p. 50.

65 Letter to author from Dr James Gray, 5 July 1996, retired City Hospital consultant, who drew these reports to my attention.

66 Letter to author from Dr Gray, 26 July 1996.

67 Gray (1999), p. 187.

68 Main (1987) 'Nursing, Midwifery and Health Visiting', in McLachlan (1987), p. 459.

69 Census of England and Wales, 1921. These rates are likely to have been underestimated as 138,211 persons in England and Wales and 841 persons in Bedfordshire failed to provide information.

70 Hardy (1993), p. 67.

71 M. Drakard (1910) 'The Nurse in Fever Hospitals', *Nursing Times*, 5 November: 906.
72 I. S. Thomson (1926) 'Children and Infectious Disease', *Nursing Times*, 7 August: 696.
73 *Burdett's Hospitals and Charities, 1930*. This hospital also had eight smallpox beds.
74 Biggleswade Isolation Hospital: Matron's Report Book, July 1929 – January 1935, and Admission and Discharge Register, January 1930 – September 1942. These records are currently held at Biggleswade Hospital, by the Bedfordshire Heartlands Primary Care Trust, who kindly granted access to them.
75 Dundas (1924), pp. 90–91.
76 Tape-recorded interview with their sister, Win Mayston (née Course), 26 April 1994.
77 Oral evidence to author, 26 May 1993.
78 Macdonald (1993), pp. 24–25.
79 Currie (1982) p. 21.
80 Ibid., p. 28.
81 Evidence from Joyce Scarlett (née Trotman), 30 July 2003.
82 L. J. Milne (1916) 'Some Points in Connection with Scarlet Fever', *Public Health*, July: 239.
83 Annual Report, MOH, Borough of Luton, 1936, p. 90.
84 C. M. Miller (1982) 'The Fever Van', *Nursing Times*, 24 March, Supplement Spotlight on Children, pp. APBN, 2–3.
85 E. V. Storey (1984) 'The Isolation Hospital at Otford in 1919', *Bygone Kent*, 5: 733–35.
86 Oral evidence to author, 26 May 1993 and 16 March 2003.
87 Ayers (1971), p. 147.
88 Ibid., pp. 34–35.
89 *BJN*, 20 December 1913: 517.
90 A. K. Gordon (1914) 'Asepsis and Fever Nursing'. *BJN*, 16 May: 432.
91 Lancet Commission on Nursing 1932, p. 235, cited in Abel-Smith (1960), p. 282.
92 Baly (1995), pp. 172–73.
93 LMA MAB, 1708A 'Nursing as a Profession', Metropolitan Asylums Board, London, n.d. [*c.*1926–27]. The putative date of this pamphlet was verified by the then, Greater London Record Office, 24 June 1996.
94 Webster (1988), p. 373.
95 Baly (1980), pp. 430–33.
96 *BJN*, May 1943: 59. Letter dated 7 April 1943, to Ernest Brown, Minister of Health, from Helena McLoughlin, Hon. Secretary, League of Fever Nurses.
97 Baly (1995), pp. 190–91.
98 NA/PRO MH55/2123 File – Proposed Closure of the Fever Register July 1952 – December 1954.
99 M. Mitman and E. M. Couzins (1953) 'Fever Training in a General Hospital', *Nursing Mirror*, 13 March: xi–xiii.
100 RCNA C337/5 Letter, dated July 1953, from Miss A. A. Ward, Matron, Neasden Hospital, London, and president of the reformed IHMNA, to matrons of the association.
101 RCNA C337. Infectious Hospitals' Matrons' and Nurses' Association: by-laws.
102 NA/PRO DT 38/34. 'Guide to the Syllabus of Examination of the Register for Fever Nurses' and Syllabus of Subjects for Examination for the Certificate of Fever Nurses, 1954, p. 15. GNC for England and Wales, 1954.

103 NA/PRO MH55/2610, GNC. Proposal to close the part of the Register for Fever Nurses – Submissions by the Council.
104 NA/PRO DT10/177, General Register of Fever Nurses, no. 5.
105 SRO GNC 12/35 Register Volume VII, Fever Part. The apparently larger number of fever nurses registered in Scotland is ambiguous, as consecutive numbers were issued regardless of the part of the Register, but the prefix E signifies the Fever part.
106 Scanlan (1991), p. 146.
107 M. Donaldson (1983) 'The Development of Nursing in Northern Ireland', unpublished DPhil. thesis, New University of Ulster, p. 179.
108 Research carried out at An Bord Altranais, Dublin in 2003, by Dr Gerard Fealy, University College Dublin.
109 Statistical analysis of the register, 1 April 2002 – 31 March 2003. The Nursing and Midwifery Council, London, January 2004.

# 4 The reality of fever nursing, 1921–71

> I do think the Fever part of the nursing profession should be kept alive, who knows what the future holds; it may be badly needed one day.
>
> Lilian Thornell (1994)[1]

## Introduction

This prophetic statement, made on reflection by a former fever nurse sixty years after she trained, recognises the value of this specialism in an uncertain world. The wisdom of years is demonstrated here, but many other revelations may be seen in the patient impact, autobiographical accounts in this chapter. They cover a broad geographical spread in Britain and the Irish Republic and spell out, very clearly, the reality of fever nursing in the period 1921–71. Moreover, they are, unashamedly, subjective in nature. Many of the all-female 127 fever nurse respondents in the study described in Chapter 1 felt strongly that 'this speciality had just disappeared' and 'had been forgotten'; 'it was an important part of nursing history' and 'their voice should be heard'. They were keen to highlight various aspects of nursing care and their training which made such a considerable impression on them that, like Lilian Thornell (née Cousins), they could still recall details, many years later.

Their testimonies are their own opinions, not those of the author. Although it has not been possible to use the data from all respondents, they provide tremendous background knowledge of fever nursing in this period. They not only convey, with devastating honesty, their feelings about fever nursing and how it affected them, but also provide an insight into the growth of antibacterial chemotherapy and, sometimes unwittingly, a glimpse of social history. Their evidence, which is too important to lose,[2] comprises the main part of this chapter and, as it confirms primary source evidence cited earlier, can mostly be taken as authentic. However, a few quite distinguished members of the nursing profession, male and female, declined the opportunity to fill in questionnaires. It is significant that they did not want it known that they had begun their careers in this speciality, or perhaps there were other personal reasons. Nurses had different attitudes to the various branches of the profession; certainly, fever nursing was seen by others in the twentieth century to be less worthy or prestigious, despite the opportunity that it afforded to learn basic nursing care and to save lives.

As has been seen, one of the differences in fever nursing was the duration and type of training. After the three Nurses Registration Acts, for England and Wales, Scotland and Ireland, in 1919, all hospital matrons in approved fever nurse training schools were required by their newly constituted GNCs to conform to a two-year standard course. The Scottish matrons did not approve and kept the third year that they favoured unofficially; nurses could then earn and receive their hospital certificate. A fever nurse course in approved hospitals could lead to a one-year reduction in general nurse training. Conversely, general nurses were entitled to a one-year reduction in fever nurse training. Even when an approved course was undertaken, its length could be extended, because sick leave had to be made up, no allowance being made for this. These facts help to explain the different periods shown after the hospital's name. Some of the eight probationers in the study, who worked in small, mostly rural hospitals, not approved for training, had clinical teaching, but there was little pretence at training. Nevertheless, they were usually awarded hospital certificates citing length of time served and their conduct; although treasured personally, they were of little value professionally.

The majority of respondents in this study entered fever nursing at 17 years of age, but following the completion of their course they had to wait until they were 20 years old before taking the registered fever nurse examination and a further year before they could be entered on the supplementary fever register of their relevant GNC .[3] Most did their 'fevers' first and then their 'general', although as will be seen, a few did their 'fevers' as a post-SRN, a one-year course, while some did no further training after their RFN qualification. Until the inception of the NHS in 1948, when practically all hospitals were appropriated by the state, most isolation hospitals, like most maternity hospitals, were managed by municipal authorities, however large or small the district. The large isolation hospitals had at least one resident physician ready to carry out a diagnosis or an emergency tracheotomy. Small hospitals were usually dependent on the local Medical Officer of Health, who was unlikely to be so readily available. However, whatever the size of the hospital, it was the nurse who was initially expected to cope in any situation.

The number of beds in any hospital was significant, in so far as it was one of the criteria for determining approval for training, but it was not always a good indicator. For example, in small rural hospitals, beds were often empty, sometimes for weeks. In epidemics they coped by, in some cases, nursing two young children to a bed, top-to-tail, opening up extra beds or using out-of-date wards and, sometimes, setting up tents in the grounds. It is clear that, apart from the theoretical component, the clinical experience gained by fever nurses was very variable. Few respondents could remember accurately the number of beds in their hospital. What really mattered was the number of beds occupied, the variety of infectious diseases and whether the necessary resources were available.

Some nurses gained experience in caring for patients who had had a criminal abortion. Before the Abortion Act, 1967, pregnant girls and women sometimes tried to procure an abortion, or get someone else, such as an abortionist, to end the pregnancy. Not only was it illegal, but also dangerous, due to lack of anatomical knowledge and aseptic technique. Those who subjected themselves to such measures could haemorrhage or become infected; both could have fatal consequences. The patient, if she survived, and the abortionist could be prosecuted. Other nurses cared for patients with pulmonary tuberculosis, because their hospital had a TB unit or a sanatorium, but this disease and the relevant patient care is not considered in depth in this book. Smallpox, and the care that was available, is covered in Chapter 5.

Before 1948, very few isolation hospitals in Britain were run on voluntary lines, unlike most general hospitals of the period. The London Fever Hospital was one of these exceptions. It was mainly supported by voluntary contributions and was originally intended to provide for paying, middle-class patients who had contracted infectious diseases. Two nurses who trained there in the 1930s set the scene for this chapter and, it could be said, the standard of care and training possible at a voluntary fever hospital then. The chapter is then subdivided in order to convey a broad cohesive picture, drawn from individual testimonials about different situations, presented chronologically, within the context of the period. The best aspects are followed by worse aspects and then night duty. Some examples of the most seriously ill patients, without identifying details, are considered next, followed by nurses who contracted infectious diseases.

The Second World War experiences and ambulance duty are included as they had such an impact on some nurses. Comparisons are then made between nurses who trained in large and small hospitals, followed by someone who trained in a large city hospital, but who subsequently worked in a small hospital. Because of its rarity value, an account is also given of a staff nurse who worked in 1938–39 in a London hospital for infants with the highly infectious disease, ophthalmia neonatorum, contracted from their mothers who had gonorrhoea. Although venereal diseases (VD) were included in the long list of infectious diseases in the fever nurse syllabus, relatively few probationers had much opportunity to nurse adult patients with these diseases, as they were mostly treated as outpatients in a special clinic. An indication of the respondents' jobs before fever nursing, and posts held after training or fever nurse experience, is then given before a conclusion is drawn. It is hoped that these carefully selected extracts convey a balanced picture of fever nursing over a fifty year period. As far as possible, the exact words of the respondents have been used, presented in a contrasting typeface, to distinguish them from the introductions which preface most sections.

## Training at a voluntary fever hospital in the 1930s

### Sarah England (Hicks), London Fever Hospital, 1933–35

I trained at this private voluntary hospital in the early 1930s. I chose this hospital as I could start nursing one year earlier than in general nursing. My GP, in

Ammanford, Carmarthenshire, knew this and recommended the London Fever Hospital. I was 17½ years old when I started training. There were about 200 beds plus about 24–30 private rooms and there was a resident doctor, Dr Massingham. I worked from 7 a.m. to 8 p.m. with three hours off duty daily, with one half a day a week and one day off duty monthly. There were two periods of three months on night duty per year. At the end of my training I was a Fever Nurse, but could not be registered by the GNC for England and Wales until I was 21 years old.

There were about 8–10 girls in my group, one left because she was homesick and found the work too hard. She was later found to have contracted TB and died the next year at home in Wales. I had a very thorough training. I was taught to help patients to be comfortable at all times and watch for symptoms – they mattered, for example, children with diphtheria might begin to choke, so we gave them plenty of pillows. I liked the company and had relatives nearby. Looking after patients was very rewarding; they were mainly children with scarlet fever and measles. There were three wards: for measles, scarlet fever and diphtheria. The private patients were mostly adults. There was also a TB ward. I found the worst aspects of training to be the fogs in London, 'pea soupers'; you could not see a hand in front of your face. I missed the green trees I was used to.

The most seriously ill patient I nursed was a young woman (33 years) with cerebro-spinal meningitis. Sister explained that her husband had to stay at home to look after their 4-year-old child. The patient had dreadful headaches, was restless and had a purple petechial rash. She was very distressed and delirious – there were no antibiotics. Her back arched, she went into a coma, had Cheyne Stoke's respirations and died. Night Sister helped me to lay her out. There were no porters, so Sister and I took her to the mortuary. The body gave frightening sighs as the last of the air was expelled from her lungs. This was my first body and experience of death which I found very distressing.

I nursed many patients with infectious diseases, including scarlet fever, and diphtheria which had a peculiar sweet smell from the toxins. I saw one child who died from diphtheria. I also cared for patients with typhoid, erysipelas, and malaria, contracted by a tea planter, who I believe was from Kenya. When he had leave he had stayed with friends in a marshy area and was bitten by a mosquito. He had dreadful rigors, but survived. I also saw a popular singer with VD. She had a terrible rash and fever with a positive Wassermann Reaction due to syphilis. The children with scarlet fever and diphtheria were in for about six weeks, but longer if they still had positive swabs. There was no visiting, except in the private wards where visitors were allowed at their own risk. They had to gown and mask up like, for instance, one visitor to a boy from Harrow School. I did not have to nurse smallpox; there was a smallpox hospital at Highgate.

The nursing textbooks we used were by Evelyn Pearce and a doctor, Handbook for Nurses by G. K. Watson. The Sister Tutor gave the Anatomy, Physiology and Hygiene lectures – the Assistant Matron, Sister Bell, gave practical nursing classes. I can't remember any doctors' lectures. I went on ambulance duty twice. I took a nurse from another hospital, who had been cared for at the London Fever Hospital, to the Brompton Hospital as she had a chest infection. The second time I went with an ambulance which brought in a lot of children with diphtheria. A doctor wanted a nurse to help with a tracheotomy in the hospital grounds and he called for a tracheotomy tray which was very quickly put together. The sisters and Matron were wonderful. The pay was £45 per annum in fevers *[higher than in other fever hospitals then].* We got our frocks and caps free, but had to buy the aprons. In general training the pay was only £30 per annum.

### Marjorie Banham, London Fever Hospital, 1937–38 (post-SRN)

The Hospital had 150–200 beds. Night duty was 8 p.m. – 8 a.m. (3 months altogether). I started training at 23 years of age following state registration. I found the other nurses, both SRNs, and students, 16–18 year olds doing a two-year course, often before general training, agreeable to work with – we saw little of Matron, but she was pleasant when we did. Our uniform was the usual cap, frock and apron; gowns, masks and gloves were available as required. I was never ill, but I think those who were received adequate attention. I do not remember any nurse 'catching' an infectious disease from a patient. We were given anti-diphtheritic serum for our own protection and were well fed, compared with what I have heard about some general hospitals.

There was a typhoid epidemic in Croydon in 1937 and we had the 'overflow' from there, but each patient had two private nurses. Although we made citrated milk, apple purée and barley water on night duty for the most seriously ill patients, we did not see them! The London Fever Hospital had a very large cubicle block and consequently a number of patients were admitted suffering from minor infectious diseases, which we would not normally have seen because they were students living in hostels, overseas visitors and others, who for various reasons, could not be nursed at home. I remember whooping cough, erysipelas, measles, rubella and chickenpox plus a diphtheria carrier, but the most common were scarlet fever and diphtheria. There was also a terminal pulmonary tuberculosis block of middle-aged men. None died while I was there, neither did the children with diphtheria, nor one young man with polio who was in a Drinker artificial lung.[4]

We did not have any textbooks; our lectures were given by Miss Clara Bell, the Sister Tutor. One good thing was that once patients were admitted, the diagnosis confirmed by Doctor Massingham and treatment ordered, he did not come to the wards unless sent for, that is, we 'nursed' the patients without the daily round of doctors one experienced in general hospitals. Usually, Dr Levine (I think), the Pathologist came when we needed a doctor – not often. I think neither he nor Dr Massingham worked such long hours as present day doctors [August 1995], but one of them was always there when we wanted someone.

One last story – I became an examiner for the General Nursing Council for England and Wales in 1967 and was approached to see if I was willing to take part in the Final Fever Practical Examination for three re-entrants to the Fever Register in the London area.[5] I was the only examiner in this area who had not previously seen these three girls, apart from my co-examiner, Miss Bell from 1937! She was very feeble physically and suggested that she examined them in theory while I took the practical exam – a suggestion I welcomed as I had not done any fever nursing since my own training, but there were practical situations common to both examination requirements. The London Fever Hospital was a 'Voluntary' Hospital, not a council one. Consequently its Doctor was not compelled to admit patients in excess of the normal bed occupancy, so we nurses did not suffer the effects of the autumn and winter epidemics, and when we had seriously ill patients, extra staff were engaged to 'special' them (see Appendix 4.5 for Miss Banham's hospital certificate).

## Best aspects

The nurses whose comments are given here show a very positive approach to their training; they were clearly keen to learn. It is apparent that the benefit which new drugs, and the use of immunisation against diphtheria, had on their patients' conditions made a great impression. They emphasised the importance of high standards of nursing care, took a pride in keeping cross infection rates low and rejoiced in new friendships. Above all, they had job satisfaction in seeing most of their patients recover, and go home.

### Annie Mytton (Elsmore), Isolation Hospital, Cheslyn Hay, Staffs, 1929–31

Matron and the senior staff nurse gave excellent personal training. All tuition was individual and nursing was to a high standard. Matron ruled with a rod of iron, but there was very little cross-infection and most patients fully recovered without antibiotics or immunisation. Numerous babies with diphtheria required tracheotomy and steam tents – most survived.

### Winifred Chapman (Bishop), North Western Hospital, Hampstead, 1936–37 (post-SRN)

The variety of experience, new drugs such as M&B revolutionised treatment of puerperal fever; Prontosil was new.[6] We had oxygen tents for 'whoopers' *[whooping cough]*, and one iron lung! We saw many cases which we did not nurse, such as anthrax, typhoid and polio.

### Rosebell Spencer (Rogers), City Hospital, Aberdeen, 1936–39

On the mixed infection ward, barrier nursing was essential. One in four babies had ophthalmia neonatorum – admitted with it – contracted during birth from mothers with gonorrhoea. Their eyes had to be bathed every four hours . . . one was made to feel responsible for the future eyesight of each child. On the second night, Sister told me that they were trying out a new drug. Treatment had been started at 10.00 a.m. and was to be repeated every four hours. This was my first introduction to M&B; imagine the joy of seeing those same eyes at 6.00 a.m. with scarcely a spot of pus! It was sheer drama. The introduction of M&B dramatically changed the treatment of infectious diseases. The Matron, Miss Frater, was a woman of great understanding and compassion; most nurses gave of their best. Discipline on the wards was strict, the educational standards high; basic nursing procedures were of prime importance. The nurses' sitting room was where we could talk freely and get rid of many irritations – a wonderful therapy!

### Kitty Bowen (Hughes), City Isolation Hospital, Cardiff, 1938–42

Most patients were very seriously ill – children mainly c.3 months – 10 years, the only drugs available at that time were M&B. Feeling content at the end of every day knowing you had contributed to each child's recovery. There was satisfaction from seeing patients recovering and going home after a long isolation period. I like to think that the good nursing they received went a long way to achieve such success. The experience of working with happy young colleagues and the friendship we had with one another.

### Barbara Cox, King's Cross Hospital for Infectious Diseases, Dundee, 1943–46

During my three years I saw the effect the use of sulphonamides had. One year later penicillin, and with the immunisation of children against diphtheria, we saw the beginning of the end of that dreaded disease, with only one ward open, as opposed to three or four when I started. I remember a 2-year-old boy with meningitis – very ill – had penicillin intravenously – little hope of his recovery.[7] We had to hold him down to give the penicillin, but fortunately he made a good recovery.

### Helen Ross (Meek), Hawkhead Fever Hospital, Paisley, 1949–52

Comradeship, meeting new people, forging lifelong friendships; caring for people – the joy of making them well again; being in almost on the ground floor of many exciting new drugs: sulphonamides, penicillin and streptomycin.[8] My certificate (RFN) was to me, from a working-class home, a passport to a whole new way of life with the potential of a profession, which, as a child, I never dreamed of.

### Elma Cooke (Petrie), King's Cross Hospital for Infectious Diseases, Dundee, 1952–55

Thorough grounding in bedside nursing. The importance of personal and patient hygiene. Lectures, some I can still partially remember. One Sister Tutor was one of the best I have ever heard.

### Olive Stewart (Stone), Northern Ireland Fever Hospital, Belfast, 1962–64

Good sound nursing care skills which have stood the test of time. In 1962 there were few nursing aids, such as special beds/mattresses, hoists, drip counters, or a central sterile supply. Care of pressure areas was meticulous. Infusion rates had to be worked out by counting the drops per minute. Instruments were boiled at ward level and then stored. The cross infection rate was very low.

## Worst aspects

The hard work, long hours and strict discipline often left nurses physically exhausted and mentally drained. Emotionally, the experience of nursing very ill children and seeing some patients die affected nurses greatly, while the apparent lack of consideration for nurses' needs was often taken personally. Of course, their comments have to be set against those stated previously in 'best aspects'; in fact, many of the respondents did not mention any worst aspects.

### Frances McCreight (Hamilton), Purdysburn Fever Hospital, Belfast, 1935–38

Seeing children choke and die with diphtheria; going to the mortuary; not always being allowed to voice your opinion about different matters.

### Alice Thorburn (Norman), Isolation Hospital, Ipswich, 1941–43

If you were on a scarlet fever ward and were told to change to the diphtheria ward at 7 p.m. to go on night duty at 8 p.m., we had to bath, wash our hair and change clothes in an hour. A bit thick if you'd had your hair permed that day!! We weren't allowed to complain!!

### Joan Mills (Wade), Marland Isolation Hospital, Rochdale, 1943–46

Many left training for various reasons – objected to the discipline; I liked it, but did not like communal life in the nurses' home. They objected to having to be in their rooms for 10 p.m. – lights out at 10.30 p.m. Very low rates of pay. Many found the work emotionally upsetting as fever nursing involved mostly young children.

### Mary Vass (Greaney), Park Hospital, Lewisham, 1946–48

Risks of infections due to exposure, long hours, severe discipline; not a happy atmosphere. My lasting memory of fever nursing was to some extent the 'FEAR' of contracting any of the diseases. At that time antibiotics were slowly coming on the scene and were making their mark. So much depended on prevention as the uptake of immunisation was very low, hence a whole ward of diphtheria.

### Audrey Goodship (Lofthouse), City Hospital for Infectious Diseases, Bradford, 1949–50 (left before finals)

Our daily chores of sweeping, dusting and cleaning were not wonderful, but accepted. Pity that in those days it was not considered valuable to just spend time with the patient. We always had to be working. Sometimes we just cleaned and tidied for the sake of it! A great source of irritation was always being unable to plan ahead for off-duty activities, since the rotas were never finalised until the last day of each week. All student nurses were obliged to live in the nurses' home where petty rules were also irritating at times; room inspected daily, including drawers and wardrobes, but no great problem.

### Barbara Dando (Milne), City Hospital, Aberdeen, 1952–54 (1955, Staff nurse)

It was so cold in the TB wards with beds out on the verandahs in all weathers. We had to put mackintoshes over the beds when it rained or snowed and refill hot water bottles throughout the night. I hated measuring the contents of sputum mugs.

### Jean Bell (Hall), West Lane Fever Hospital, Middlesborough, 1955–57

Deaths in young and small children; looking after septic abortions, and VD. Seeing a dead foetus. Doing loads of sluicing and emptying mugs from TB patients. Seeing children upset when relations could just look through windows at them when visiting.

### Jean Castleton (Old), West Lane Fever Hospital, Middlesbrough, 1965–67

Having to treat the Consultant as though he was God, and the sluicing of all the nappies, previously soaked in diluted Izal for 12 hours.

## Night duty

Night duty is included because so many nurses felt that it was a particularly trying time. In the period discussed here, 1924–59, it was common practice in many fever hospitals, particularly the smaller ones, to have only one nurse on night duty, who was sometimes on 'sleeping duty', that is, available to answer a call. Although this practice may have developed management skills, young, inexperienced nurses often felt vulnerable and were sometimes at risk – as were their patients. In large hospitals the Night Superintendent, or Night Sister, usually visited up to three times to offer advice and support, but they were not instantly available in an emergency. This was also custom and practice in many general hospitals in the same period, as was the manner in which these (mainly teenaged) probationers were often informed that they were to go on night duty, which frequently appears to have been peremptory and lacking in consideration.

### Anne Rogerson (Gloag), Lightburn Fever Hospital, Glasgow, 1924–27 (Figure 4.1)

I was on night duty on a 50 bed ward, alone. Barlinnie Prison was next door. In about 1925 there was an outbreak of diphtheria. The prisoners were sent to our fever hospital, therefore, we were locked in at night with them. Not one touched you – they were very helpful in the mornings, except one man who seemed quite quiet. He threw a cup of tea over me. There was an awful lot of cleaning, no hoovers or polishers, and the discipline was terrible, like being in the army.

### Violet McGhie (Thompson), Joint Hospital, Dumbarton, 1929–30 (did not complete)

I don't know how nurses in that line of work survived as it was really slavery. As a very early probationer I helped to take a body to the mortuary, where I had to get up on the table to light gas mantles, lay out white sheets on the table and hold them straight – this at nearly midnight.

### Annie Mytton (Elsmore), Isolation Hospital, Cheslyn Hay, Staffordshire, 1929–31

Having to be on call every night. Sleeping in a room between two wards – this had a window where we could observe the patients. We had to get up when they called. I had to move between wards of diphtheria and wards of scarlet fever patients with only a white gown for barrier nursing. Wards were mixed – men, women and children together; seriously ill patients with those convalescing.

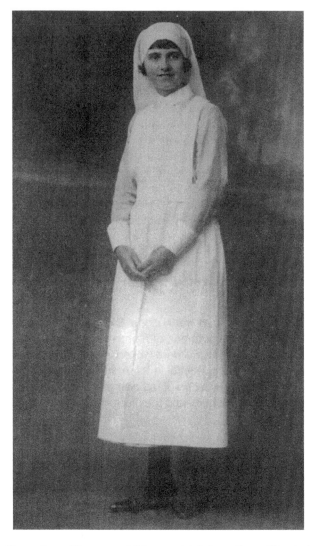

*Figure 4.1* Nurse Anne Gloag, aged 18 years, Lightburn Fever Hospital, Glasgow, 1924. Courtesy of her son, Mr Kenneth Rogerson

### Elizabeth Cunningham, Musselburgh Fever Hospital, Edinburgh, *c.*1934–36

As it was a small hospital there was no night nurse unless there was an epidemic, which we had once or twice, of scarlet fever, otherwise there was always a nurse who did 'sleeping duty' in a bed in the duty room! There were only 30–40 beds – staff: Matron, one Sister and two probationers.

### Winnie Anderson (Alexander), King's Cross Hospital for Infectious Diseases, Dundee, 1936–39

Changing from night duty to day duty, we left the ward at 2 a.m. to start again at 7.30 a.m. Likewise, coming on night duty from days, we were called to start work at 2 a.m.

### Mair Williams (Davies), Hill House Hospital, Swansea, 1937–41

I still remember the suffering of fever patients. I pray future generations won't become apathetic re immunisation. All blanket bathing was done during the night, females one night, males the next night. We started at 2 a.m. Apart from Ward 2 (diphtheria), where there were two nurses on duty, a staff nurse and a probationer, there was only one probationer on each ward.

### Peggy Crisp (Tomkins), Isolation Hospital, Over, Gloucester, 1937–41 (1942, Staff nurse) (Figure 4.2)

We worked long hours in those days, half day off each week, one whole day a month, for 30 shillings [£1.50] a month. On night duty we had two shifts off a month, one nurse per ward (often 20–24 patients), no meal breaks, some toast or a sandwich eaten in the ward kitchen. We were all very happy, loved the work and our companions, the only grumbles I remember were about lectures at 10 a.m. after night duty, aching feet and being so tired (we also had air raids to contend with). We borrowed clothes for dates, shared goodies from home – they were very happy days.

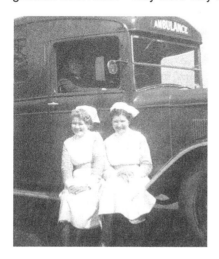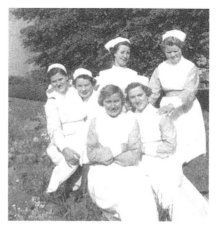

*Figure 4.2* Nurses off duty at Over Isolation Hospital, Gloucester, 1939–40. Peggy Crisp (née Tomkins) front right in group. Courtesy of Mrs Beryl Nobbs, sister of the late Peggy Crisp

### Barbara Doran, Fazakerley Fever Hospital, Liverpool, 1944–45 (post-SRN)

Fazakerley was believed to have 1,800–2,000 beds, the next biggest to Monsall at Manchester. It was divided into blocks with spacious grounds between. As it was so big, four Matrons did their rounds by bikes between the blocks. A student nurse had to move the bike from one end of the ward to the other, so it was ready for Matron to get back on when she had completed the length of the ward. There were always two nurses on night duty per ward.

### Annie Dearden (Cowie), Ruchill Hospital, Glasgow, 1950–52

Too much responsibility too early in training. After less than six months, first year probationers were left in charge of wards (on night duty). The majority of us were still less than 18 years old! Tubercular meningitis was treated at this time with streptomycin and PAS.[9] As a direct result of the streptomycin, quite a number of our patients were deaf. This caused a great deal of distress.

### Bridie Hartley (Geraghty), Dublin Fever Hospital, 1957–59

Night duty on isolation wards – trying to attend to 20 or more patients in individual cubicles on my own. Sluicing and disinfecting dirty sheets before sending to the laundry. Some of the ward sisters were very difficult to work for. Lifting polio patients with paraplegia up in bed without help. No such thing as 'lifting techniques'. Probably, why I now have back problems!

## Most seriously ill patients

In the section on 'Best aspects', nurses recalled with pride those who recovered. Here death dominates, particularly young death. It is clear that this was an aspect which disturbed them. Many years later, some nurses could still recall their very ill patients' names and other details, although not given here. The number of deaths quoted here could be confirmed in local MOH or county MOH annual reports, but the more statistically correct rates were seldom given. Neither was it common practice in the years cited here (1924–55) to compare mortality rates between different fever hospitals as there were too many imponderables. It would have been highly contentious and those found to be deficient would probably have had to close, leaving some areas without any provision. In many cases, where patients were seriously ill, particularly before immunisation was in common use and prior to the advent of antibiotics, it was often the high standard of nursing care which made the difference between life and death.

### Anne Rogerson (Gloag), Lightburn Fever Hospital, Glasgow, 1924–27

Diphtheria patients dying like ninepins – nine out of ten children died. More deaths from this than any other disease. There were no inoculations then, they were only just coming in. We had to apply linseed oil poultices half-hourly for our pneumonia patients; the hot oil eased their breathing.

### Lilian Thornell (Cousins), Little Bromwich Fever Hospital, Birmingham, 1932–33 (post-SRN)

A girl, aged 4 years, with measles – neglected at home – admitted with septic corneal ulcers. In spite of intensive treatment, she lost the sight in both her eyes. Two girls aged 7 years, both at the intravenous stage of diphtheria; one from a good country home died. The other from a slum house in Birmingham recovered. Who had the most immunity?

### Gwyneth Badham (Rees), Tumble Isolation Hospital, Llanelli, 1935–37

I distinctly remember a 12 year old with diphtheria (bull-neck) getting better, then dying after six weeks with heart failure.

### Bridget Rafferty (McCaughey), Ruchill Hospital, Glasgow, 1936–39

Most of the patients were very ill – diphtheria of all ages, but mostly children; severe typhoid in adults; poliomyelitis, all ages; tubercular meningitis, usually in very young children. Children and adults with pneumonia; it was severe as there were no antibiotics at that time. A large amount of tracheotomies were done in diphtheria. We had severe typhoid patients. We also had undiagnosed black sailors from overseas, usually via Glasgow docks.

### Effie MacDonald (MacAskill), City Hospital, Edinburgh, 1942–45

My first ward was TB – there were 12 deaths in the three months I was there, most of them young people.

### Alice Williamson (Jackson), Western Hospital, Fulham, 1943–45

An RAF Pilot Officer contracted poliomyelitis nine weeks after getting his wings. He was nursed intensively in a Drinker's apparatus, but he died c.1946, aged 21 years.[10]

### Marjorie Tobyn (Le Gry's), Myland Hospital, Colchester, 1943–46

My first experience of infantile paralysis, a young woman of 30–40 years who could not move, and would lie with tears running down her face. She died.

### Stella Baird (Hall), Purdysburn Fever Hospital, Belfast, 1944–46

The day before discharge from scarletina, a 4-year-old boy developed tetanus, from a cut from a seaside bucket, and died; a 16-year-old school-boy, with a broken neck from a rugby injury, died in an iron lung; four service-men, paralysed due to sulphonamides being injected into the spinal canal instead of by intra-muscular injection at an army hospital, and many young women who died from TB meningitis before penicillin.

### Dora Deacon (Goodwin), Borough Isolation Hospital, Burton-on-Trent, 1944–46

There were no drugs in those days for tuberculosis. Some recovered, but many died. It was just 'general nursing care'. Most were fairly young, 20–30 years old. Occasionally, there were old patients, probably up to 50 years.

### Anne Lawrie (Edgar), Hawkhead Infectious Diseases Hospital, Paisley, 1949–52

Patients dying from tuberculosis, mostly young people; septic abortions – one woman died aged 28 years, and the small children who died from TB meningitis.

### Mary O'Shea, St Finbarr's Hospital, Cork, 1951–52 (post-SRN)

We had some typhoid patients. In the 1950s, some Spanish fishermen used to go along the seashore and pick up shellfish while their boats were in port.

### Elma Cooke (Petrie), King's Cross Hospital for Infectious Diseases, Dundee, 1952–55

I particularly remember: Weil's Disease, the child recovered; poliomyelitis, an 18-year-old nurse from Dundee Royal infirmary, who recovered, but was left in a wheelchair; tuberculous meningitis, a 55-year-old woman who died after two years and a 30-year-old male who contracted typhoid fever from work abroad – he recovered.

### Barbara Dando (Milne), City Hospital, Aberdeen, 1952–54 (1955, Staff nurse)

During the 1950s there was a great deal of poverty in Aberdeen. Our hospital was very close to the slum area. The mortality rate amongst babies, I would say, was pretty high. They used to come in with gastro-enteritis, malnutrition and rickets. We had quite a few regulars – a lot of them died too. In 1952, a male dock worker in his 30s caught Weil's Disease. I found it very harrowing; he died. During the poliomyelitis epidemic in 1955 there was a high incidence of death in all age groups.

## Nurses who contracted infectious diseases

As was seen in Chapter 3, it was not unusual for nurses caring for patients with infectious diseases, to contract such diseases themselves, either from their ward, or from outside the hospital. Some, apparently, had had no previous exposure to a particular disease or had a poor immune response. The following extracts have been selected to illustrate how some nurses were affected.

### Dorothy Martin (Bass), North Eastern Fever Hospital, Tottenham, 1921–23

When the ward was very busy there was no time for a meal. I, therefore, got run down and contracted scarlet fever. Occasionally, other nurses caught diseases. At such times, scarlet fever and diphtheria were nursed on the same ward. There was very little cross-infection.

### Violet McGhie (Thompson), Joint Hospital, Dumbarton, 1929–30 (did not complete)

I took a bad throat, saw my GP – he took a swab for diphtheria – it was clear, but he advised me to give up infectious disease nursing.

### Iris Gordon (Westcott), Grove Hospital, Tooting Grove, 1936–38 (1939, Staff nurse)

Of the 50 nurses in my group at the beginning of training in 1936, only three did not finish – one died from diphtheria, one married and one returned home – homesick.

### Bridget Rafferty (McCaughey), Ruchill Hospital, Glasgow, 1936–39

One of my friends developed typhoid; she was extremely ill, but recovered. She lost all her hair, but as a bonus it grew in curly. She completed her training. A good number of nurses developed scarlet fever. I left Ruchill with a shadow and scarring on my left lung, but was unaware of this; I was unable to continue my training at the Middlesex Hospital after being X-rayed for superannuation.

### Elizabeth McLean (Grieve), City Hospital, Edinburgh, 1938–41

Probably the worst thing in my training was a really bad dose of scarlet fever which I took after four months, followed by jaundice, and later that year a positive swab for diphtheria, but it was very mild. In 1939 I got pneumonia; I was very poorly and was treated with linseed poultices and M&B 693.

### Margaret Gorman, Purdysburn Fever Hospital, Belfast 1939–40 (post-SRN)

I had anti-diphtheria vaccine on starting the course but caught a mild attack which left me a carrier. I had to have my tonsils removed before I could get the three consecutive negative swabs necessary for my discharge.

### Ursula Cork (Watts), Brook Hospital, Woolwich, 1939–42

My training was extended by six months as I caught scarlet fever, mumps, rubella and hepatitis.

### Dorothea Furber (Hammond), Isolation Hospital, Davenham, Cheshire, 1939–42

The reason for my training lasting more than two years is that I contracted measles at the end of my first year – we didn't have anyone in hospital with that, but my fellow pupil, who was the same age as myself [17 years] also contracted measles and we passed it on to all the children in the scarlet fever ward. Whilst making up the time that I had been off with measles, at the end of October 1941, I contracted diphtheria in spite of being immunised at the start of my training.

### Alice Williamson (Jackson), Western Hospital, Fulham, 1943–45

Very few nurses caught infectious diseases – they were routinely warded and then returned to duty. Sadly, quite a few died of pulmonary TB including an Indian girl and Irish nurses coming from country areas to London. My feeling is that they did not catch it from their work. I caught mumps from my young sister whilst at home and was blamed for the outbreak that followed on the ward.

### Jane Day, City Hospital, Edinburgh, 1943–46

I remember a few nurses who developed TB and some left after contracting diphtheria. I caught diphtheria in about 1946. We had a test for scarlet fever called a Dick test; also one for diphtheria, the Schick test. That year I had been overlooked for the Schick and caught the disease. I was nursed in the hospital (all nurses were treated as private patients and nursed in cubicles on a separate ward). I was off work for three months, happily with no lasting damage.

### Jane Tivnann (Devine), Strathclyde Infectious Diseases Hospital, Motherwell, 1957–60

About 1958, one of my colleagues contracted tuberculosis. She was nursed for a year at Strathclyde Hospital.

### Yvonne McKinley (Austin), Northern Ireland Fever Hospital, Belfast, 1969–71

Some staff occasionally contracted diarrhoea and vomiting or head lice, but nothing ever very serious.

## Second World War experiences

Fourteen nurses in this study were, to a greater or lesser extent, affected by problems in or surrounding the Second World War. For some there were real hazards; others who trained in this period (1939–45) were apparently left unscathed as they failed to mention the war as an event significant to them. The war gave them the opportunity to meet patients from different surroundings and different nationalities, sometimes with tropical diseases. Penicillin was mainly available only to service personnel, but it is clear that some fever patients were given it due to the medical staff knowing someone who had access to this new 'wonder drug'.[11] Necessity maximised the use of penicillin. Many of the typical social disruptions of war are illustrated here, including the abandonment of unwanted infants. Despite overwhelming tiredness at times, these nurses, buoyed up, perhaps, by their youthful vigour and sense of patriotism, seemed to take most of the adverse situations they met in their stride.

### Ruth Brend (Gleeson), Little Bromwich Fever Hospital, Birmingham, 1939–40 (post-SRN)

During the air raids of 1940 the Hospital was hit by incendiary and high explosive bombs, but although the laundry, kitchen, Maids' Home and a cubicle block were damaged, there was only one minor casualty.

### Peggy Crisp (Tomkins), Isolation Hospital, Over, Gloucester, 1937–41 (1942, Staff nurse)

In 1940 we had a very large diphtheria outbreak due mainly to the children not being immunised and in the shelters at night. At one time we had two small children in the top and bottom of a bed, mostly 4 and 5 year olds. I remember also being sent to special several tracheotomies, the old sterile feather procedure[12], no sucker then. Drugs were also rather limited, M&B 693, Streptocide, Prontosil and anti-diphtheria toxin. Penicillin was first used in 1942 as an orange powder, perhaps I should say crystals. Mrs Ethel Florey, wife of Howard Florey, was experimenting on different types of infection at the Central Middlesex Hospital. I used to trail up to the Path Lab with Winchesters full of urine for the excreted penicillin to be extracted and given back to the same patients. It was in very short supply.[13] Cetavlon also came out that year, and the non-touch technique for dressings.

### Edith Boardman (Green), Isolation Hospital, Rush Green, Romford, 1938–40

Due to air raids we returned to cooking our meals on the wards on night duty. When an air-raid siren shrieked, we usually took up a position under an empty bed. We were dead tired and so slept and often did not hear the 'all clear'. When the gardeners were called up we formed a rota to care for the grounds.

### Margaret Chaffer (Swanston), City Hospital, Edinburgh, 1938–41

We nursed under very difficult conditions in wartime – respirators having to be manually worked in underground shelters.

### Mary McFarlane (McWilliams), City Hospital, Edinburgh, 1938–41

We did a bit of nursing service personnel during the war – patients with influenza and pneumonia, mostly Navy, when we opened more wards.

### Ursula Cork (Watts), Brook Hospital, Woolwich, 1939–42 (1946–53, Staff nurse)

When the air raids started we had to nurse the babies on a mattress underneath their cots. Some patients were nursed in the corridors in sleeping bags as this was considered safer, our hospital being surrounded by military establishments. Next door was the Royal Herbert Military Hospital, in addition there were barracks, anti-aircraft gun sites and, of course, Woolwich Arsenal. We had our share of high explosive bombs, incendiary bombs and two rockets, some on the Hospital and some in the grounds. Often patients would have to be moved to other wards, all in semi-darkness, lit only by the fires started by incendiary bombs. When dawn came and the bombers were gone, who was most exhausted, those who had been on night duty or those in air-raid shelters who had had little sleep, if any, and had to drag themselves on duty at 7.15 a.m.?

Three porters were killed in cellars under the wards; they were on fire watch duty. Two doctors were also killed elsewhere. Nurses slept in different cellars under the sun terrace of the nurses' home, although they were reluctant to do this. Home Sister sought them out from under their beds or in wardrobes and sent them to cellars which were infested with mice and where five nurses had to sleep on two mattresses on the floor. In the 1942–43 raids, and later in the war, no patients or nurses were killed. One unexploded bomb fell in the grounds, but the only injury from this was when a bomb disposal man fell into the deep crater and broke his nose!

### Lillian Ewins (Boyle), Brook Hospital, Woolwich, 1939–41 (Enrolled nurse 1946)

As the war was coming we had to take the overflow from the military hospital next door. Half of the Brook was fevers, the other half general. Missing sleep due to air raids and having to go on night duty again during the night was terrible. My friend, Ursula Watts, and I used to stand on a bridge between the two nurses' homes and watch the Battle of Britain Spitfires coming back from a raid doing victory rolls in the sky. We took the casualties from the bombing, along with the local children with infections. Although we were allocated a ward, we were moved according to urgent need at the time. One day would be a general ward, another would be de-lousing children who had been sleeping in shelters, or looking after babies that had been abandoned. There was a ward full of healthy babies who had been left in churches, on doorsteps or on Woolwich Common.

After she left, by now married and having had a baby at the Brook in 1942, Lillian remembers the direct hit on the Medical Superintendent's house. His wife, who had organised a dinner party, and another doctor were killed. Two ward blocks (A and B) were bombed. One porter was killed but, she believes, no patients or nurses. By then the hospital had stopped using the upstairs wards and sandbagged the ground-floor wards. When bombs were falling, cots were wheeled into the corridors away from flying glass.

### Dorothea Furber (Hammond), Isolation Hospital, Davenham, Cheshire, 1939–42

For me the war meant having to get up when the sirens went, carrying the children to the shelter, 'sleeping' with them until 5 a.m. and getting up again at 7 a.m. We had a variety of what today, would appear to be minor infections, due to the evacuation of many poor children from Manchester and Salford to large country houses in the vicinity, and also the billetting of many soldiers on large country estates nearby.

### Olive Dodd (Cowley), Dunstable and District Joint Isolation Hospital, 1942–44 (Figure 4.3)

At Christmas 1941, when I was a patient with scarlet fever, every bed was occupied, so children were nursed two to a bed, top to tail. I became a probationer there at the age of 17 years in 1942. Epidemics sometimes affected whole families or a group of children from a class. Boys from Dunstable Grammar School, who were boarders, and soldiers from the town barracks were admitted during the war. This was one reason why patients were rarely homesick as, once recovered from the initial serious stages, they began to recognise familiar faces around them. Visitors were not permitted inside the wards; they usually came only on Sundays, but could see very little as the

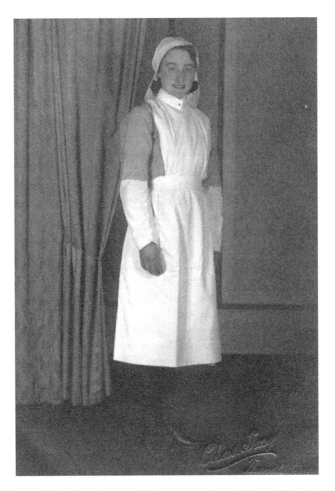

*Figure 4.3* Nurse Olive Cowley, aged 17 years, at Dunstable and District Joint Isolation Hospital, 1942. Long sleeves of uniform dress were removed for practical work. Courtesy of Mrs Olive Dodd

windows were protected by sandbags. Restrictions on time and rationing of food were accepted as a normal part of wartime life, with strict discipline enforced as it was in the services. Off duty was spent helping on the land, tending the rhubarb and vegetables, but everyone particularly enjoyed picking apples in the orchard and laying them on shelves in an outbuilding ready for use throughout the winter.

It was usually one of the probationers who took it in turns to do night duty, running between the three blocks in complete darkness due to 'black out' precautions. She decided her base, dependent on the location of the youngest or illest patient. Fire watching was also carried out during the night. When there were only a few convalescent patients I did 'sleeping duty'. This involved settling the patients for the night, retiring into a camp bed under the scarlet block stairs, relaxing sufficiently to undo my collar stud and hopefully, sleeping until morning *(see Appendix 4.7 for Mrs Dodd's hospital certificate)*.

### Alice Williamson (Jackson), Western Hospital, Fulham, 1943–45

During my training, the very first married nurses were accepted, mainly married to servicemen, who were tidily out of the way. One, however, was pregnant and kept on night duty – eventually she was allowed to leave her belt off.

### Flora Milne (Todd), King's Cross Hospital for Infectious Diseases, Dundee, 1942–45

I nursed two servicemen, one Polish man who died from tuberculosis and one Naval Officer who died from polio.

### Effie MacDonald (MacAskill), City Hospital, Edinburgh, 1942–45

There was an outbreak of meningitis in Dreghorn Army Camp; ten young men and all went out cured.

### Stella Rose (Waters), Infectious Diseases Hospital, Colchester, 1944–47

There were no male nurses in training, but we did have male orderlies from the army.

### Christina McGregor, Burgh of Motherwell and Wishaw Infectious Diseases Hospital, Motherwell, 1945–48

One of the saddest cases I specialled was an ex-Japanese prisoner of war, a 24-year-old male, the last death from diphtheria I tended. In 1945 the local authority became Labour. The Council introduced, generally, a 48 hour working week (the first in the UK). Shifts had to be introduced 7–3; 3–11; 11–7. Two weeks were allocated on each duty at a time, with a day off weekly. Their next act was that we were required to join a trade union. We rebelled and the Royal College of Nursing eventually accepted it, after a long dispute but no strike. Therefore, we had a 48 hour week, a night duty shift of 8 hours and six weeks' annual leave. *[Most fever hospitals continued split shifts until closure.]*

## Ambulance duty

The need for a nurse to accompany patients with infectious diseases to hospital was not recognised universally in Britain until the early twentieth century. Before the inception of a rudimentary land ambulance service in 1881, run by the Metropolitan Asylums Board, and its river ambulance service on the Thames in 1884 in London,

> Nurses to accompany the sick were seldom provided; in most cases the patient travelled alone, and occasionally reached the hospital dead or in a dying condition. Sometimes the patients were accompanied by friends, not always sober, who returned home in public conveyances. The MAB therefore thought it necessary, that an experienced nurse and a male attendant, to help the nurse carry patients over 10 years old, accompany each ambulance. Fever nurses were allocated from the adjoining hospital on a daily basis; there was, therefore, always a nurse in readiness for a call.[14]

This system did not prevail everywhere. Dr A. K. Gordon, Lecturer on Infectious Diseases at the University of Manchester in 1914 (previously Medical Superintendent of Monsall Fever Hospital), recalled a situation in *c.*1901, when he saw an ambulance arrive at a certain hospital loaded with three children from different houses packed in with some filthy bedding. Although the children had been notified to the Sanitary Authority as cases of scarlet fever, this was not so, as, on examination, one was found to have diphtheria. They had travelled to the hospital without even a nurse.[15]

Nurses travelling in horse-drawn ambulances, particularly in remote rural areas in other parts of Britain, could be subjected to a relatively long journey away from their hospital, during which their patient's condition could deteriorate. Food and stimulants were commonly provided for patients. For example, by 1907, a nurse always accompanied the ambulance when it was sent to fetch a new patient for admission to Cork Street Fever Hospital, Dublin. She carried an emergency bag which contained stimulants and before she left the patient's home gave a handout of published information to the relatives, which included how to make enquiries about the patient.[16] The MAB horse-drawn ambulances were last used on 14 September 1912. 'The familiar sight of urchins shouting "fever!" was lost on the London scene'.[17] Well into the twentieth century, the sight of the fever van, whether horse drawn or motor driven, still caused excitement for bystanders and dismay for patients, which could cause problems for the accompanying nurse. Edith Webb, a young girl in early-twentieth-century Luton, recalled in 1993, seeing the van with yellow wheels from the municipal Spittlesea Isolation Hospital in the terraced streets of the town.[18] In 1994, a man still remembered from his boyhood seeing the distinctive royal blue Daimler ambulance reserved for patients being transported to the fever wing of Clayponds Hospital, South Ealing, in the Second World War.[19]

Eventually, most isolation hospitals, whatever their size, sent their probationers out on ambulance duty in their own ambulance kept specifically for cases of infectious disease.[20] Although larger hospitals with many admissions could allocate nurses on a planned basis, smaller hospitals used a more *ad hoc* system. The GNC for England and Wales included details of nursing care and treatment in the transport of infectious patients, in the Record of Practical Instruction and Experience for the Certificate of Fever Nursing under 'Special Experience'.

Textbooks for nurses contain additional sources of information about ambulance duty, showing the important part it played in nursing care and nurse training. For example, *Fevers and Fever Nursing* by Evelyn Pearce includes Final State Examination questions for five years, 1935–1940. Question 3, in February 1935, shows the depth of knowledge required and the responsibilities given to probationers:

> What are the duties of a fever-ambulance nurse? State in detail what steps you would take if the patient appeared to be dying
> (a) on your arrival at the house, and
> (b) in the ambulance on the way back to hospital.[21]

Joyce Watson, another Sister Tutor, explained in detail what was expected on ambulance duty. Nurses were to act on special instructions, but 'occasionally to exercise their own discretion'. The patient's doctor or their own authority could be telephoned in case of difficulty. As the ambulance nurse was the first and, perhaps, only representative of the hospital, she should be courteous, considerate and dignified. A detailed case history had to be obtained and children under 7 years of age labelled. The patient was to be wrapped in blankets and carried to the ambulance. The nurse could ask the driver to proceed more quickly, or slowly, if necessary. Water, brandy, a feeding cup, swabs and sanitary utensils should be available for the journey and the vessels cleaned between cases. Once at the hospital, the receiving room nurses helped transfer the patient to a bed or couch. Having checked the history together (out of the patient's hearing) the doctor was called to examine, diagnose and dispose of the case.[22]

Apart from one fever nurse probationer at Liverpool, who was already an SRN and, therefore, over 21 years of age, the following nurses were impressionable young women, about 17–20 years of age, used to the hygienic surroundings of a clinically clean hospital where they did as they were bid, seldom using their own initiative. On ambulance duty it was different.

### Glenys Rees (Hickman), North Western Hospital, Hampstead, 1934–36

I very much enjoyed the experience of going out on ambulance duty – I saw so much of the home life, especially the poverty in which some children lived. Also seeing the 'sights of London' was a nice change from duty!

### Elizabeth Cunningham, Musselburgh Fever Hospital, Edinburgh, 1934–36

The ambulance was horse-drawn and we felt very important in our uniforms and cloaks when out with the driver admitting the patients. Everyone in the town knew when a patient was going to the fever hospital.

### Peggy Crisp (Tomkins), Isolation Hospital, Over, Gloucester, 1937–41 (1942, Staff nurse)

On our off-duty hours we were often asked to go out on the ambulance to fetch a patient. We did not mind at all, it was a nice change and saved taking a nurse off a busy ward.

### Elizabeth McLean (Grieve), City Hospital, Edinburgh, 1938–41

We all had a term of ambulance duty when we went out in the hospital ambulance to pick up the patient that had been notified. If you felt there was any question of the diagnosis being incorrect, you had the ambulance stopped at the main office and asked for a doctor to look at the patient, rather than risk cross-infection. If a laryngeal diphtheria was notified we went with sirens sounding both ways. Sometimes a doctor came with us and if need be did an emergency intubation or even a tracheotomy in the ambulance. It's been known for laryngeal diphtheria patients to die in the ambulance. I always remember being sent out . . . for a case of erysipelas of the face, but it didn't look right, so of course I asked for a doctor. This lady was isolated in a side ward and diagnosed as anthrax. She was a florist and was thought to have got it from infected straw used to pack flowers from the Channel Islands. She died about ten days later.

### Mary McFarlane (McWilliams), City Hospital, Edinburgh, 1938–41

One case is very much in my memory, sixty years later. A little girl with diphtheria had not been notified to the City Hospital as being an obvious case; she was coming from a hospital outpatient department (OPD), so we collected a possible case of diphtheria first and then went to OPD as it was nearer our hospital. When I saw the child I informed my escort that she was dying and we shouldn't take her, but was ordered by the doctor to do so. We ran with her and her mother, but she died in my arms a few minutes into our return journey – a horrible experience. My Chief exonerated the ambulance crew and myself. What happened afterwards we never found out. She had not been immunised and nothing would have saved her really as Mother was probably even too late taking her to OPD. Sticks in my memory though.

### Ruth Brend (Greeson), Little Bromwich Fever Hospital, Birmingham, 1939–40 (post-SRN)

The hospital ran its own Ambulance Service with a nurse always in attendance. Our role in collecting patients was to examine the sick person and write up a synopsis of the condition and the symptoms presented. I remember bringing in a soldier with Vincent's Angina; he was very ill but did make a good recovery. Another case I collected was an airman with cerebral – spinal meningitis; he too recovered. I think I learnt more about fevers whilst on ambulance duty because of the variety of diseases.

### Dorothea Furber (Hammond), Isolation Hospital, Davenham, Cheshire, 1939–42

If a patient needed admission, the first person Matron met in the nurses' home, from the appropriate ward, was volunteered to go on Ambulance Duty, and we covered quite a distance.

### Madeline Foster (Tovey), Borough Isolation Hospital, Burton-upon-Trent, 1942–43 (did not complete, State Enrolled Assistant Nurse later)

It was the duty of a nurse to go with the ambulance to pick up patients. Tracheotomies were quite common in cases of diphtheria. We were instructed how to perform one in an emergency and to keep the hole open until the tube could be inserted. These were cleaned with feathers in those days.[23]

### Olive Dodd (Cowley), Dunstable and District Joint Isolation Hospital, 1942–44

One of the most interesting nursing duties was to accompany the Infectious Diseases' ambulance, partly to coerce the patient into being admitted, but also (as it was wartime) to collect the gas mask, ration book and bedding. At one house, eight evacuee children slept on the floor on heavily soiled mattresses which obviously needed fumigating. As only one child was to be admitted, the foster mother was naturally reluctant to part with the communal bedding. Arguments at some houses had to be resolved by the Police who intervened when requested.

### Barbara Doran, Fazakerley Fever Hospital, Liverpool, 1944–45 (post-SRN)

I usually picked up deprived, malnourished children from slummy areas like Upper Parliament Square and Scotland Road. We were not always very welcome. I also went to ships to collect servicemen, especially a group of Canadians from a transit camp in Canada who had an outbreak of mumps. No drugs were given by nurses on ambulance duty until the patient was seen by a hospital doctor.

### Jeanette Walker (Gunns), West Lane Hospital, Middlesbrough, 1945–49 (trained 1946–48)

We used to go out in the ambulance to collect our patients. Children used to collect near the ambulance and hold their noses so they wouldn't 'catch the fever'.

### Olga Henderson (Smallman), Hospital for Infectious Diseases and Grindon Hall Sanatorium, Sunderland, 1946–48

I went out for patients as a student nurse. I wore a white coat and mask. Sometimes, I went to houses where patients had already died. What do I do now?

### Lilian Miller (Barnsley), Strathclyde Infectious Diseases Hospital, Motherwell, 1953–55

I saw the poverty when we went out to houses to collect patients and we nursed a lot of neglected children.

## The large versus the small hospital – a comparison

Conditions for patients and staff in large and small hospitals were often very different. Large hospitals were more likely to be staffed by experienced RFNs and nurses in training for that qualification, whereas small hospitals often relied on one RFN and young women who did not have an opportunity to train for a recognised qualification. Some examples are, therefore, given of five nurses who trained in large fever hospitals between 1936 and 1955, followed by four who worked in small fever hospitals between 1931 and 1953.

## Large fever hospitals

### Sarah Donnelly (Brooks), Grove Hospital, Tooting Grove, 1936–38

Our Sister Tutor, Miss White, made our lectures so interesting. It was fascinating to learn of the special horses whose serum was obtained from their jugular veins for diphtheria. A scratch on a calf's abdomen produced serum for smallpox; anti-snake serum was obtained from snakes at London Zoo, and leeches were acquired from a farm in Wales; they were removed from the skin by tweezers.

### Joan James (Mills), City Fever Hospital, Birmingham, 1937–39

There were 1,000 beds. All the nursing staff, medical officers and domestic staff had excellent Homes, as everyone was resident and full time. There were bedrooms and recreation rooms, a library, writing rooms, laundry, tennis courts and a ballroom with a stage for staff shows, which were performed by each group about twice a year; there were also dances. The dining room was staffed by uniformed resident staff, resembling a dining room in a three star hotel. There were two, or sometimes three, sittings of four meals and a snack at mid-morning, when everyone took a clean gown on duty for that day. The food was excellent, a well-balanced diet; very little sickness among staff. There was a sick bay in the nurses' home which was well equipped under the charge of two home sisters, with a doctor in attendance when called. Nurses' salary was £2 per month, uniform provided. Off-duty was three hours a day, two half days a week and one day a month. We did six months on day duty and then six months on night duty – on duty twelve nights and three nights off. Sleeping-out passes were issued from Matron's Office. We had two weeks' annual leave with pay.

### Dorothy Millard (Arnold), Grove Hospital, Tooting Grove, 1938–40

I found the training excellent in every respect. We had a wonderful tutor and our schedule was methodically kept up to date. Although The Grove was a LCC Hospital, the training was superior to that which I received later at a voluntary hospital for general training, but we did not have a library; that would have been an asset.

### Jeanette Walker (Gunns), West Lane Hospital, Middlesbrough, 1945–49 (trained 1946–48)

I knew the difference (by smell) of scarlet fever, diphtheria, tonsillitis and other diseases. Everywhere was scrupulously clean, open windows, sunshine and Izal. We had to wear masks, gloves and gowns when giving streptomycin, which TB patients bought privately from the USA.[24] They lived outside on verandahs. We had to run round with macs to put over their beds when it rained and thaw their drinking water when it froze. Took me in at 16, as I wanted to be a nurse, and laid out my first dead body at 16.

### Sarah Kelly, Strathclyde Infectious Diseases Hospital, Motherwell, 1953–55

The best part was the bedside nursing, hard work, but great job satisfaction. There were high standards. Very few patients were 'up and about'. Fever nursing gave me a very good grounding in basic nursing care and observations, that is, always observing the different stages of each disease, complications and effects on patients; my ward organisation and managerial skills began in 'Fevers'. I did enjoy the theoretical aspect of my training which was planned on the Block System. We also had to attend a weekly test in school.

## Small fever hospitals

### Eve Saddington (Richmond), Holly Lane Fever Hospital, Smethwick, 1931

It was not a training hospital and when I realised I was wasting my time and no qualification could be won I left. I was 17 years old. I then started as a student in a hospital for 'mental defectives' and gained the certificate of the Royal Medico-Psychological Association (RMPA).

### Ella Cross, Guisborough Isolation Hospital, Cleveland, 1933–35

I trained at Guisboro' Fever Hospital for two years. It was newly built and I was the first nurse employed there. No written qualifications were given. There were probably two wards and six cubicles. We had no specific hours of day duty. On night duty you were alone; the hospital was isolated under the hills – very frightening. Off-duty was when you could be spared. Quite a number of children died from diphtheria. The Sister or Matron were called when this happened on night duty. There was a Matron, a Sister and three nurses in total. I loved the work I was doing. I nursed patients with diphtheria, quite a number died; scarlet fever, chickenpox, erysipelas and puerperal sepsis. There were no textbooks; I bought an Honnor Morten dictionary and a Nursing Mirror pocket encyclopaedia. During my two years there I contracted diphtheria and scarlet fever.

### Dora Deacon (Goodwin), Borough Isolation Hospital, Burton-on-Trent, 1943–46

I started as a 'sub probationer' aged 16 years in 1943 at our local fever hospital. It was too small to take the RFN certificate, but we had lectures, an examination and a hospital certificate after two years training.

## Jill Forder (Stott), Spittlesea Isolation Hospital, Luton, 1952–53

I was a nursing cadet for fifteen months at this non-training hospital which was near Luton Airport and Vauxhall Works. I remember Spittlesea well and the experience it gave me for my general nurse training at the Luton and Dunstable Hospital. Looking back, it is quite horrifying the responsibility given to me at 16 years of age. I was left in charge of patients with polio', iron lungs, tiny babies in oxygen tents, the Lysol scrubbing of hands and drug control – duties way beyond my skills. There were many staff,[25] including Sister Tibbles, who was the RFN there, Sister O'Farrell and Nurse Jones; they gave me such a good grounding for my career. I worked three different shift patterns: 7.30–5.30 p.m., 11.00–8.30 p.m. and 8 p.m. to 8 a.m. There was no training programme for me, but I could learn from those already trained – the basic nursing and isolation techniques from that era. Most of the patients who died were infants with multiple pathology. The polio' patients were mostly young adults, some of whom survived in this pre-Salk era;[26] children, 4–16 years with lesser complications recovered. I also nursed patients with other diseases: diphtheria, scarlet fever, whooping cough, measles, mumps, rubella, chicken-pox, glandular fever, syphilis, salmonella, erysipelas and bacillary dysentery. Most people have forgotten that fever nurses existed, yet it was fascinating at that time, especially experiencing the changes since then.

Relatively few fever nurses in this study worked in both large and small hospitals and were, therefore, unable to comment on the varying standards. One exception is given in the example which follows.

## Ruth Brend (Gleeson), Little Bromwich Fever Hospital, Birmingham, 1939–40 (post-SRN) and Bucknall Fever Hospital, Stoke-on-Trent, 1940–41

I was 22 years old when I went to Little Bromwich. There were six in our set of SRN fever trainee staff nurses, five of us completed, one having left to get married. There were three resident doctors for, I believe, 900–1,000 beds. Little Bromwich Fever Hospital, was, in my opinion, very up-to-date by the standards prevalent in 1939. It was at that time run by the Public Health Department of Birmingham City Council. Bucknall Fever Hospital was, by comparison, antiquated. During my year as a ward sister there I experienced nursing of an epidemic of typhoid fever. There were 60 plus cases, with ages ranging from 1–60 years. Two obsolete wards were opened up to accommo-date the patients, one for males and the other for females. Unlike Birmingham, there were no sterilisers for bed pans and utensils and all excreta had to be treated with disinfectant before disposal. The only means for heating drinks for the patients was an old-fashioned kitchen range – which we, as nurses, had to keep alight with coal. Birmingham's rule was that no food or drink could be consumed by the staff on the ward, but in Bucknall the nurses were expected to cook on an antiquated kitchen range and eat on the ward at night.

## St Margaret's Ophthalmia Neonatorum Hospital, Kentish Town

Ophthalmia neonatorum was made a notifiable disease in February 1914. It is a very serious condition, contracted during birth from mothers with gonorrhoea, affecting the eyes of newly born infants, which may result in permanent blindness. It requires special treatment and isolation. Following an order from the Local Government Board in 1917, the MAB opened an institution known as St Margaret's, in Leighton Road, Kentish Town, London, on 16 September 1918. By 1929, about 150 mothers and 250 infants were being admitted annually, only one-third of all notified cases in London. Venereal diseases are not, and never have been, notifiable diseases. Nevertheless, the MAB opened a hospital for patients with these conditions, the Sheffield Street Hospital in Kingsway, London on 21 June 1920.[27] St Margaret's and Sheffield Street Hospitals seemed to have worked together with maternity hospitals in London for women with VD. As a result of the Local Government Act, 1929, the London County Council assumed responsibility for St Margaret's and Sheffield Street Hospitals in 1930, which then had, respectively, 60 and 52 beds. The testimony of a nurse who worked at St Margaret's in the late 1930s follows.

### Winifred Chapman (Bishop), St Margaret's Ophthalmia Neonatorum Hospital, Kentish Town (1938–39)

Following three years' general training, 1933–36, I qualified as an RFN in 1937 after a one year course at the LCC North Western Hospital, Hampstead; I then did midwifery training. In 1938, I went to St Margaret's, a very small hospital for women with gonorrhoea or syphilis, and infants, toddlers and young girls with ophthalmia neonatorum. It existed until the outbreak of war in September 1939, when it was evacuated.[28] The nursing staff consisted of Matron, three sisters, one staff nurse with general and midwifery certificates (me), two trained staff nurses and a number of assistants. I was almost the youngest there.

There were three floors: the lower floor had 12 beds for mothers transferred from maternity hospitals in the London area, some of whom were transferred to Sheffield Street Hospital in central London; some babies were alone. The middle floor had toddlers and small children – I had very little to do with them. The top floor was mostly for girls in care from remand homes; they had daily treatments. They had to do all the cleaning on their ward, not enough to keep them occupied. Twice a week a woman came to teach them sewing. They hated it. I relieved on all floors. I remember more about the infants. The few married women, mainly failed prostitutes, were allowed husbands to visit (very few of them). I was responsible for the mothers' daily treatments such as douches and occasional eye treatment for the babies. I remember it was a solution of Eusol and they had hourly or two hourly washouts for their eyes. As result of this, the babies did not thrive; they got little rest. They were fed on Nestlé's milk as the visiting doctor was very keen on this, which did not suit many babies; they were very sickly.

In the year I was there only one baby became blind, most responded to treatment well. The eye surgeon was Mr Cadell. We did get some trainee eye nurses and visiting nurses for lectures. I was there until the outbreak of war, and was evacuated with babies and some mothers to a hospital for the mentally deficient in Swanley, Kent. Other patients were sent to various places. I resigned in October 1939 and have no idea what became of the hospital. No one seems to have heard of St Margaret's. My salary was £80 yearly, plus £5 for midwifery certificate, plus £90 living-out allowance. I was rich. I married and gave up nursing. I am 81 years old now *[1995]* and have an excellent memory.

## Career pathways

The total number of respondents was 127, all female, 109 of whom (86 per cent) gained a registered fever nurse qualification or its equivalent. They trained between 1921 and 1971 in all parts of Britain and in the Irish Republic:

| | |
|---|---|
| England | 61 |
| Wales | 1 |
| Scotland | 32 |
| Northern Ireland | 12 |
| Irish Republic | 3 |
| Total | 109 |

Number of respondents who did not gain a recognised qualification: 18. Reasons given:

| | |
|---|---|
| Not a training school | 8 |
| Reasons associated with the Second World War | 4 |
| Left before finals | 2 |
| Left to get married | 1 |
| Dismissed by Matron in 1939, with three colleagues, for going out after finishing duty at 8 p.m. | 1 |
| Left after receiving hospital certificate | 1 |
| Ill health | 1 |
| Total | 18 |

## Jobs before fever nursing

Number of respondents who stated their job before fever nursing: 39 (31 per cent) of the 127 respondents. This was not a compulsory question. Some left school at the age of 14 years, so they needed to find other work before taking up nursing. Although some were already state registered nurses, or held another registerable qualification and were, therefore, over 21 years of age, others were quite young, 16–17 years of age, when they were employed in a caring capacity. Various euphemisms for job titles were used in hospitals partly to disguise the fact that they were, perhaps, taking advantage of youthful enthusiasm, which often put them at risk of contracting infectious diseases. The jobs cited are in the exact words of the respondents.

| | |
|---|---|
| Shop assistant | 4 |
| Farm work | 1 |
| Children's nurse | 1 |
| Live in nanny | 1 |
| Care of baby with cleft palate and sewing-room work in a factory | 1 |
| Children's ward in isolation hospital | 1 |
| Residential night nurse | 1 |
| Nursing home | 1 |
| Cadet nurse | 4 |
| Pre-nursing school | 3 |
| Nursing assistant | 2 |
| Sub-probationer | 2 |
| Ward orderly | 1 |
| Training began at 16 | 1 |
| Assistant nurse | 1 |
| Junior trainee residential hospital nursery | 1 |
| State registered nurse | 3 |
| Began SRN, did not complete | 2 |
| British Tuberculosis and Thoracic Association (BTTA) | 2 |
| TB sanatorium | 1 |
| SRN and Registered Sick Children's Nurse (RSCN) | 1 |
| RSCN | 1 |
| SRN and State Certified Midwife (SCM) | 1 |
| SRN and Central Midwives Board, Part I | 1 |
| Orthopaedic Nursing Certificate | 1 |
| Total | 39 |

## Posts held after training or fever nursing experience

Although this was not a compulsory question, of the 127 respondents, 111 (87 per cent) answered. As many worked in a number of situations, wherever possible, their ultimate post has been quoted; their answers have been categorised into sections. The 13 RFNs with a single qualification had varied experiences when the fever registers closed at about the same time as some isolation hospitals. Some were allowed to transfer, or convert, to another two-year course, not the three-year SRN course, and this only if supported by nurse management. They could not then hold, for example, the RFN and the enrolled nurse qualification. On principle, the holding of two statutory qualifications from one training period was not permitted by the GNC.[29] In some enlightened general hospitals, where there was a separate isolation unit in which they were employed, their jobs were protected and they were still treated and paid as staff nurses. Some fever nurses gave up the struggle to convert, often because they had not carried out any study recently; others chose to work as nursing auxiliaries or nursing assistants, but one left the profession, feeling disgruntled. Certainly, the single RFN qualification limited career progression.

*Hospitals: 51*

| | |
|---|---|
| Sister or staff nurse in: | |
|    a general hospital | 17 |
|    a fever hospital | 10 |
|    own fever training hospital | 9 |
|    a child isolation unit in a general hospital | 6 |
|    an ophthalmia neonatorum hospital | 1 |
| Management in a general hospital | 4 |
| General nursing, responsible for control of infection | 2 |
| Management in isolation hospital | 1 |
| Management in a children's hospital | 1 |

*Midwifery: 3*

| | |
|---|---|
| Sister or staff nurse | 2 |
| Enrolled nurse | 1 |

*Private sector: 13*

| | |
|---|---|
| General nursing | 9 |
| Industrial nursing/occupational health | 4 |

*Community: 10*

| | |
|---|---|
| Public health, including health visitors | 5 |
| School nursing | 2 |
| Management | 1 |
| Health visiting and school nurse | 1 |
| Cottage hospital | 1 |

*Other specialisms: 10*

| | |
|---|---|
| Nurse education | 3 |

| | |
|---|---|
| Practice nursing | 3 |
| Psychiatry | 1 |
| Mental subnormality ward sister | 1 |
| Management | 1 |
| Radiotherapy centre | 1 |

*Armed services: 5*

| | |
|---|---|
| Queen Alexandra's Imperial Military Nursing Service in | |
| England and India | 3 |
| Africa | 1 |
| Queen Alexandra's Royal Naval Nursing Service | 1 |

*Other work abroad: 2*

| | |
|---|---|
| Tanganyika General Hospital | 1 |
| Matron, College in Malaysia | 1 |

*RFNs with single qualification: 13*

| | |
|---|---|
| 'Transferred' from RFN to state enrolled nurse | 6 |
| Nursing assistant, hospital or community | 4 |
| Nursing auxiliary | 2 |
| 'Not allowed to convert' | 1 |

*Jobs outside nursing: 4*

| | |
|---|---|
| Trained as a primary school teacher | 2 |
| Shop assistant | 1 |
| Nursery nurse | 1 |

## Conclusion

The eyewitness accounts in this chapter have, by virtue of their consensus views on different aspects of fever nursing in the period 1921–71, provided for the first time a broad profile of the reality of this, now almost forgotten, speciality. The 127 respondents were a self-selected sample yet, despite the variables, they have greatly contributed to the body of knowledge in the history of nursing. Two trained in a London voluntary fever hospital, where they were, to a certain extent, protected from seriously ill patients, thereby missing some clinical experience. Neither were they overburdened with work in epidemics, as funds were, apparently, readily available to employ extra staff, and to provide a higher salary for their fever nurses than in other isolation hospitals.

The 8 nurses who worked in small, non-training hospitals and the 117 who undertook a recognised fever nurse course were employed in municipal hospitals managed by their local authority until 1948. Even then, fever nurses were, until the closure of most isolation hospitals, and the professional registers in the late 1960s and early 1970s, because of the living-in requirement, a ready source of labour, useful in epidemics. However, living-in provided a sense of camaraderie, a familiarity when friendships could develop. There was a sense of trust which boded well when wards were hectically busy; teamwork was easier. Calmer periods were experienced when most patients were convalescent. Nevertheless, it was a cloistered environment, almost like being in a closed religious order, particularly for those in small, remote, rural hospitals where social opportunities were less likely and nurses were almost as isolated as their patients. Wherever they worked or trained, they were employees, never truly student nurses.

The emphasis was on service needs, rather than on education, although for those on approved courses, there was a recognised curriculum with the number of hours in practice and theory laid down, which had to be completed. Admitted, almost always as young women, 16 to 17 years of age, they were moulded into obedient, knowledgeable beings and encouraged to become general nurses. Planned allocations, if they existed at all, could be disturbed by the urgent need for another nurse on a particular ward, or even a sudden change from day to night duty. However, fever nursing developed their powers of observation; most probationers could recognise different rashes and differentiate one disease from another by a distinctive smell, especially diphtheria. Not all hospitals included ambulance escort duties but, when required, probationers welcomed it for the novelty factor and because they recognised that it broadened their professional knowledge and awareness of social conditions. It also enabled them to use their own initiative (as on night duty) instead of merely obeying orders, frightening though this was at times, because of their age and inexperience.

The evidence presented, taken from their testimonies, could be seen as contradictory, particularly in the best and worst aspects of training. It is clear that they are personal perceptions of what was right and proper and what was reasonable when they trained, mostly acceptable then, but sometimes questioned later on reflection. For example, the importance of hierarchy and hospital routine, even carrying out bed baths from 2 a.m. onwards, apparently obediently and without question, but strict rules as regards eating in the ward could be waived when circumstances changed. The long hours and strict discipline, with often unquestioning obedience to authority, was mostly accepted by these respondents. Few of those who demurred appear here.

Common threads throughout these testimonies have been the need to accept change and adapt to different circumstances, exemplified by nurses in the Second World War. Earlier methods of nursing care, such as the application of stupes (compresses) and poultices, gradually gave way to reliance on antibiotics. Each in their turn, the sulphonamides, penicillin and streptomycin, were witnessed with a sense of wonder for their, mostly positive, effect on seriously ill patients – a sense of relief that recovery was now more likely.

However, some also saw the serious side effects of new drugs such as streptomycin, and witnessed the harm caused when sulphonamides were given by the wrong route. Sagely, they also noted the benefit of immunisation against diphtheria; when effective campaigns were carried out in the community, diphtheria wards could be closed.

The prominence given to hygiene and the strict measures taken to prevent cross-infection was another theme as was the, at times, devastating exposure to death – very often in young children. However, none of the respondents used the term 'stress' and none stated that they were formally counselled. In fact, the view was that 'talking it over in the nurses' home' relieved their anxiety; it provided catharsis, closure. They accepted that contracting infectious diseases was 'par for the course'; none complained, perhaps because the need for absence from duty provided a break, although, they commented ruefully, they had to extend their training period. Most respondents agreed that fever nursing, where high standards of hygiene and basic nursing care were learned, was an excellent foundation for general nurse training. Youthful vigour and enthusiasm, a devotion to duty which, at times, bordered on the heroic, shine through many accounts. They may have been exploited by management for their labour, but working and training in large fever hospitals gave them the opportunity to become professional nurses.

## Notes and references*

1 Lilian Thornell (née Cousins), Little Bromwich Fever Hospital, Birmingham, 1932–33 (post-SRN) in a letter to author, 8 November 1994. Lilian, then 86 years old, was reflecting on her early days in fever nursing.

2 All the papers from the 127 respondents, and other relevant documents, will be deposited in the Royal College of Nursing Archive in Edinburgh.

3 In the Irish Republic the qualification was registered infectious diseases nurse.

4 The first mechanical respirator to be used widely was named after Philip Drinker, an engineer working at the Harvard School of Public Health in 1928. For details see Gould (1995), pp. 90–92.

5 As the Fever Nurse Register closed in England and Wales in December 1967, this was probably their last chance.

6 Prontosil, a sulphonamide, available from *c.*1936, greatly reduced mortality from puerperal (childbed) fever. In 1938, May and Baker (M&B) developed M&B 693, another 'sulpha drug', even more effective against this fever and other streptoccocal infections.

7 Penicillin, discovered by Alexander Fleming at St Mary's Hospital, Paddington, London, in 1928, was not ready for use until the Second World War. Although initially used for service personnel, it was used for civilians later in the war.

8 Streptomycin, discovered in 1943, by Selman Waksman, an American microbiologist, was obtained in pure crystalline form in 1944.

9 Para amino salicylic acid.

10 See note 4.

*————

Full references appear in the Bibliography.

11 K. Brown, 'Fever Nursing' (personal communication by email, 30 June 2003). Mr Kevin Brown, Archivist of St Mary's Hospital, Paddington, London, and author of the biography of Alexander Fleming (Brown, 2004), who discovered penicillin there in 1928, confirmed that this information was substantially correct. He stated, that 'apart from personal influence in obtaining the drug, which shouldn't be discounted as I have seen evidence that the system was bucked in order to obtain it for patients, it was also possible to obtain it through approved channels for selective clinical trials. By 1944/45 there was an official regional distribution system to which application had to be made for any use of penicillin and for access to supplies'.

12 The sterile feathers were delivered to the ward in a packet and were autoclaved, along with the dressing drums, the night nurses had to pack in those days.

13 Kevin Brown (personal communication: see note 11): 'Ethel Florey was indeed conducting clinical trials at the Central Middlesex Hospital. Penicillin would have been powdery rather than crystalline. The recycling of penicillin from urine is attested, first at Oxford with Florey and Fleming's first systemic case, and then later at other hospitals'.

14 LMA MAB 1686, 'The MAB of London and its Work', 1900. See also Ayers (1971), pp. 188–89.

15 *BJN*, 9 May 1914: 409.

16 Scanlan (1991), p. 109. See also Figure 2.6 on p.29.

17 Ayers (1971), p. 189.

18 Oral evidence to author, 4 January 1993.

19 Recollection of Mr Ronald Smith to author, 26 September 1994.

20 Until 1948, municipal hospitals, such as those for infectious disease patients and maternity patients, usually kept their own ambulances on site, while other hospitals and infirmaries generally used those run by the police.

21 Pearce (1940), p. 271.

22 Watson (1945), pp. 5–7.

23 See note 12.

24 See note 8.

25 Other local isolation hospitals closed or changed their use soon after 1948, including Dunstable and District Isolation Hospital which, from 27 January 1949, became known as the Priory Hospital and started to admit pre-convalescent, geriatric and chronic sick patients. In February 1950, Letchworth Isolation Hospital was converted into a children's convalescent home. By March 1950, Spittlesea Isolation Hospital, Luton, catered for South Bedfordshire, part of North Hertfordshire and took all cases of poliomyelitis from North Bedfordshire. The hospital was particularly busy in the early 1950s with a polio epidemic, but it was able to recruit extra nursing staff, including some from isolation hospitals which had closed.

26 The Salk vaccine was named after the American virologist, Jonas Edward Salk. His vaccine, which could be given orally, used a killed polio virus, unlike the Sabin vaccine, which had to be injected. For more detailed information, see Gould (1995).

27 Ayers (1971), pp. 184–85, 274–75. Ayers gives 1917 as the opening date of St Margaret's (p. 185), but in the main data given on p. 274, the date is given as 1918. According to *Burdett's Hospitals and Charities, 1919*, p. 325, this hospital was established in 1918 with 30 beds for infants and 18 for mothers. The Matron-housekeeper was Miss E. Mearns. Ayers also gives a succinct summary of how the LCC worked to provide facilities to prevent the spread of VD under the Public Health (Venereal Diseases) Regulations, July 1916.

28 Winifred Chapman believes St Margaret's was never used as a hospital again.

29 See Chapter 8, 'The single qualified nurse' section.

# 5    Smallpox nursing

> Few diseases have been so destructive to human life as smallpox, and it
> has ever been regarded with horror alike from its fatality, its loathsome
> accompaniments and disfiguring effects, and from the fact that no age or
> condition of life are exempt from liability to its occurrence.
>
> *Black's Medical Dictionary*, 1916

## Introduction

The general public and most nurses in practice now have little knowledge or
experience of smallpox, despite its fearful reputation, and yet the history of
smallpox nursing provides lessons which have immediacy in the twenty-first
century. The threat of biological warfare is a very valid reason for learning
from the past. This ancient disease, properly termed variola to differentiate
it from the great pox (syphilis), had been endemic in Britain since at least
the fifteenth century. It became more prevalent from the mid-1660s after
the decline of the plague and, therefore, the most feared of the pestilential
diseases. It bears a 30 per cent case-fatality rate but, in confluent smallpox,
it can be as high as 50 per cent. There is no treatment. Between 1851–60 and
1891–1900, the mean annual national mortality rate of deaths due to smallpox in England and Wales declined considerably from 202 to 13 per million
persons living.[1]

Some serious epidemics of the more dangerous form of the disease, variola
major, the severe Eastern type, still occurred, the worst being in 1870–72,
1884–85, 1893–94 and 1901–02. Major epidemics of variola minor (alastrim),
the milder Western form, occurred in 1928–29 and in 1947 and there were
other outbreaks from time to time, all of which were to have implications for
modern nursing care as the profession developed. As there was no cure for
smallpox, the introduction of vaccination, discovered by Edward Jenner in
1796, the first preventive measure against any infectious disease, was of major
importance. It gradually replaced the more hazardous practice of inoculation,
which protected by inducing a mild fever and, sometimes, a serious form of
the disease which could be transmitted to others. Inoculation could also result
in the inadvertent transmission of other diseases, such as syphilis. Public

health measures, were implemented throughout Britain, yet the disease was not declared eradicated by the World Health Organisation (WHO) until 1980, the last known case being in Somalia in 1977.[2] However, stocks of the smallpox virus are held under properly controlled conditions in freezers in Moscow and Atlanta[3], despite reservations by some epidemiologists.

The disease itself has been the focus of considerable research. An extensive archive already exists, including the work of Edward Jenner (1749–1823),[4] but there is, as yet, no seminal work on smallpox nursing in Britain, probably because the evidence is scanty and scattered. Sources for this chapter include official reports, diaries, books, journals, newspapers and testimonies from those who nursed patients with the disease.[5] The knowledge which emerges could be useful for nurses and others involved in the event of what is now termed 'biological terrorism'. Germ warfare experts acknowledge that the smallpox virus is 'the most dangerous and potentially devastating of all weapons'.[6] In 1980, the likelihood of accidental or deliberate release of smallpox from a laboratory was regarded, by the United States, as 'close to nil',[7] despite the case of Janet Parker, a British photographer working above a research laboratory in Birmingham in 1978, who died after contracting the disease through the ventilation system.[8] There is also historical precedence for 'bioterrorism'. In the pre-vaccination era, during the French and Indian Wars in North America (1754–67), British soldiers distributed blankets used by smallpox patients, thereby deliberately causing outbreaks among the American Indians, which resulted in a 50 per cent mortality rate.[9]

Smallpox could once again threaten the nation's health because of an ill-advised, wilful action elsewhere. Current international concern has now been aroused as stocks of the smallpox virus, in addition to those properly deposited, are probably being concealed by Iraq, North Korea and Russia. Moreover, for some years, the Soviet Union has researched ways of genetically altering the virus. The importance attached to these actions may be seen by the following reactions. The first national symposium on the Medical and Public Health response to Bioterrorism was convened in February 1999, in Arlington, Virginia: forty-six states and ten countries, including Australia, Canada, Britain, France, Germany and the Netherlands were represented.[10] The City of London Police Force disclosed in August 1999 that senior officers had been trained in command procedures necessary to respond to chemical/biological terrorist incidents and England held its first national conference on the subject in October that year; twenty-three countries sent delegates.[11] Nurses are mostly unaware of how vital they, and other health care workers, would be in the event of an outbreak of smallpox.

Smallpox, caused by a brick-shaped virus, was spread mainly by droplet infection to very close contacts, by bodily contact, through fomites such as skin scales and debris from bedding and clothing and, possibly, by aerial convection. Transmission did not occur during the ten to twelve day incubation period. The disease had a sudden onset with the development of a high temperature with severe muscular pains, often with severe backache, nausea and vomiting which lasted for two to four days, before the eruption of the typical smallpox rash of macules, then papules, then vesicles, then pustules. The prognosis was dependent upon whether it was variola major, more common in the eighteenth and nineteenth centuries, or variola minor, which predominated in Britain after 1901.[12] The outcome was also determined by the clinical type of smallpox:

- modified (mildest)      patients partially protected by an earlier attack or vaccination with, therefore, only a small non-pustular eruption
- discrete      manifested by individual pocks which remain separate
- confluent      very profuse rash, with the spots coalescing to form large blebs. Temperature does not fall to normal when the rash appears, as in mild cases.
- malignant (haemorrhagic)      blebs filled with blood instead of serum. Bleeding also occurs from all orifices and some organs; death commonly ensues within the first week.[13]

Those who survived could be permanently disfigured by scars from deep pockmarks. They were usually much deeper and more disfiguring than those left as a result of chickenpox. Some people also lost their sight. Fashionable ladies in the eighteenth century sometimes covered stigmatising pocks on their faces with black patches, a craze often taken up by others who had not been affected. However, for the nation, the implications of an epidemic were more serious because it diminished the population, locally and nationally and was, therefore, a threat to the nation's economy, a point often mentioned by officials and doctors throughout the period when outbreaks occurred, but rarely by those involved in the direct nursing care of the sick.

Smallpox was mostly regarded as a disease of the poor, who were more likely to contract it because of their crowded living conditions, but the well-to-do were not immune; for instance, Queen Mary II died of the disease in 1694,[14] and in France, King Louis XV succumbed to it in 1774.[15] Until the mid-nineteenth century, children were more commonly affected than adults. The reasons for this are not clear, but it may have been the result of the Vaccination Act, 1853, when the vaccination of infants, before they were 4 months old, became compulsory.[16] As the care of patients with smallpox by professional nurses did not generally begin in Britain until the late nineteenth century, this chapter focuses initially on an earlier period, when the majority of the population lived in a rural environment. Sufferers were then mostly cast upon the care, or lack of it, in local communities. Patients are often said to be unseen in nursing history – not so here. It is only by considering them, and whether they were cared for at home or in an institution, that a picture begins to emerge of those who provided care. Four case histories in Britain help to illustrate this; one is also given of a British family in India in the days of Empire.

## Early nursing care in the community

Here the local example is particularly important; it highlights the lack of professional nursing in the eighteenth and early nineteenth centuries and the consequent burden on relatives and the parish, then the secular as well as the spiritual authority. In this context, the term 'nurse' is used in its broadest sense as an attendant, such as relative or neighbour, good or wise woman, and later, as institutions were established and nursing developed, a pauper nurse, an assistant nurse, a probationer or a trained nurse. They were predominantly female, but men were occasionally needed, especially for their ability to control delirious patients. For example, Stephen Blundell was paid £2 out of the poor rates of Cheam, Surrey, on 4 October 1741, for nursing Bridget Pullen with smallpox, for a fortnight.[17]

Most people relied on received wisdom, handed down to them, when caring for the sick, although books began to offer advice for the literate. John Wesley (1703–91), the founder of Methodism, knew of tried and tested remedies for different ailments through his extensive travels. His 1747 text, *Primitive Physic*, included a section on smallpox. Some measures concerned diet: 'Drink largely of toast and water: Or, let your whole food be milk and water, mixed with a little white bread: tried. Or, milk and apples'. Another suggestion, probably due to the contemporary belief that infectious diseases were spread by miasmas, perhaps due to the objectionable smell, or to combat the fever, 'Take care to have free, pure and cool air. Therefore open the casement every day: only do not let it chill the patient'. Other remedies related to the local management of pustules, and popular treatments commonly advocated in other ailments: bleeding, a gentle vomit or a gentle purge. Finally, a procedure which has survived – the changing of the sick, 'with very dry, warm linen'.[18]

William Buchan (1729–1805), the Scottish physician, expanded Wesley's wisdom in *Domestic Medicine* (1769). He observed that other children were most liable to the disease and termed those who provided care, 'good women'. He provides one of the earliest modern accounts of care, which includes a vivid description of the conditions that prevailed in London in 1769 among the poor afflicted with smallpox at home. He observed that two or three children with the disease were often lying in the same bed 'with such a load of pustules that even their skins stick together. One can hardly view a scene of this kind without being sickened by the sight'. Their linen was not changed throughout the illness. As the young patients were so often 'peevish' and refused to stay in bed, the constant presence of a nurse was necessary. Buchan also criticised the dangerous practice of crowding. He had seen, for instance, 'above 40 children cooped up in one apartment'. He recommended keeping the patient cool and quiet, and bathing the feet frequently with warm water. Suppuration should be promoted once the pustules appear by 'diluting drink, light food, and if Nature seems to flag, by generous cordials' (stimulants and tonics). The patient should be taken frequently out of bed and excessive restlessness curbed by gentle opiates 'administered with a sparing hand'. Advice was also given to the 'good women' to help them cope with care of the mouth, urinary problems and constipation. He warned that when the eruption subsides suddenly, 'the danger is very great'.[19] Victims might then receive some nursing care at home, but the tendency was to cast them out like lepers and incarcerate them elsewhere to prevent the spread of the disease.

## Pesthouses and other evidence of smallpox

During the seventeenth century, pesthouses had been established in some areas to isolate plague victims; some survived to the eighteenth century to house those with smallpox. Where none existed, and there was a need, parishes rented or built cottages. They were usually established on the edge of parish boundaries, well away from the church and most dwellings, such as the one known to have existed at Luton on the Great Moor in 1724. Dunstable also had a pesthouse at the end of West Street at the junction of the old Green Way or Drovers Way, but it was not used after 1784.[20] The overseers of the poor raised the necessary funds to maintain the sick. A number of late-eighteenth-century houses of industry in East Anglia also provided detached pesthouses for those with infectious diseases.[21]

In about 1745, a pesthouse was established at Caddington, funded jointly because it stood on the borders of Hertfordshire and Bedfordshire. The total cost, including firewood for drying out the new house, was £60 10s 0d (£60.50).[22] Articles of Agreement on 8 November 1757 refer to 'a certain House called the Pest House belonging to the said Parish of Caddington . . . for the Reception of nursing and providing for such poor Persons . . . afflicted with the Distemper called the small Pox.'[23] It was demolished in 1840 at a cost of £2 5s 0d (£2.25).[24]

The small county of Bedford is believed to have supported fifteen pesthouses in the eighteenth and early nineteenth centuries, two of which, at Leighton Buzzard and Chalgrave, survive.[25] The Chalgrave Pesthouse was established by the parish church, *c.*1797, on land which it still owns (Figure 5.1). Originally two semi-detached cottages, each with one room downstairs containing a large fireplace and stairs to the one upstairs room; they are now part of a much larger dwelling house. The well survives in the garden. It is likely that a caretaker and his wife lived in one cottage and the other was kept empty for anyone needing isolation for smallpox. However, by 1837, no longer used for smallpox, they were sold.

Pesthouses have also survived in Hampshire and at Framlingham, Suffolk. The latter was originally a two-storey house, occupied by a nurse who under-took the care of smallpox patients sent in by the parish.[26] The wife of the caretaker of the pesthouse, or neighbours, often paupers themselves, also paid under the local parochial system, sometimes provided 'care'. Which form it took is uncertain, probably just the provision of basic necessities, such as food

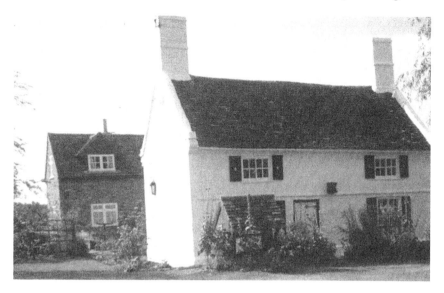

*Figure 5.1* Chalgrave Pesthouse, Hockliffe, Bedfordshire, established *c*.1797, seen in the foreground, with the original well. The Pesthouse, converted for private accommodation, is now part of a larger dwelling. Courtesy of Mr Ray Attewell

and water. However, like the smallpox hospitals established later, pesthouses usually stood empty for long periods and were not always ready when an epidemic occurred. Often, the only record that an epidemic had occurred, before civil registration of deaths began in 1837, was a note in the parish registers that a number of people had died from a particular disease. Sometimes, the only indicator was the increased number of burials in a relatively short period.[27] Such records contain no information on the provision of nursing care. Some details, however, may be gleaned from diaries because of the impact the disease had locally, at a time when individuals were all known to each other. Tombstones and memorials can provide other relevant data.

The diary of the Reverend Benjamin Rogers, Rector of Carlton, in North Bedfordshire, 1720–71, provides a unique insight into contemporary life there and in surrounding areas; matters affecting the wider world were also thought worthy of note. For example, the first entry in the edition which covers the years 1727–52 mentions that Sir Isaac Newton died in March 1727. It covers a range of issues including accidents, his own illnesses and different diseases; smallpox is mentioned four times. An entry on 23 October 1729 concerned an outbreak of a mild form of the disease at Huntingdon, and at Godmanchester, where over 200 people were affected. Only two died, and they, apparently, killed themselves. A further diary note of 29 April 1731 records the death of a Mr Thomas Carter of Turvey who died of smallpox fourteen or fifteen days from the first signs. He was buried the day after death, presumably because of the bad state of the body and the fear of contagion.[28]

Rogers was clearly dismayed about the 5 July 1736 outbreak in his own parish of Carlton, which affected five families. It was believed that it had been brought in by people from Olney, where the disease had been raging for a long time. The last outbreak Rogers referred to was in Bedford. On 18 January 1739, he noted that the Reverend Mr Francis Hunt, Vicar of St Paul's, Bedford, had died of smallpox. Although the outbreak, which had been there for a long time, had seemed mild at first, it had now developed. It 'now begins to be very bad, and a great many now die, whereas at first but very few died'.[29] Little could be done for people who contracted the disease, except wait for the outcome.

The Reverend James Woodforde (1740–1803), Rector of Weston Longville, Norfolk, from 1758 to 1803, was also sufficiently interested in his own and his parishioners' illnesses to record them in his more well-known diary. In March 1791, he described the rapid spread of smallpox in the parish and showed how small tokens of care could make a difference to those affected. He personally donated a shirt to one man to ease the discomfort caused by his own rough one, and also provided food and drink for the family. The diary shows the personal loss he felt following the death of his young carpenter, John Greaves, for whom the doctor was summoned too late. He left a pregnant wife and a small child.[30]

Similarly, a memorial of a woman who survived smallpox for fifteen years before her death in 1796 gives some indication of the physical and mental after-effects she suffered and the grief felt by her family.

> Erected by a Sister in Memory of her beloved Anna Cecilia, Daughter of Christopher Rhodes Esq. of Chatham in the County of Kent. She departed this Life, June 2$^d$ 1796, aged 32. She was the Delight of her Parents and the Admiration of all who knew her. At the Age of 17, the Small-pox stripped off all the Bloom of youthful Beauty, And being followed by a dreadful Nervous-disorder, withered those fair Prospects of earthly Happiness Which were expected from her Uncommon Affection, Sensibility and Tenderness.[31]

It is not known where or how she contracted smallpox, but Chatham, like other ports, was prone to epidemics because of diseases imported from other countries. People in Britain were at risk of contracting smallpox from travellers, particularly sailors and soldiers returning home from various wars. The largest epidemic in nineteenth-century Europe occurred when troops were demobilised at the end of the Franco-Prussian War in 1871.[32] Residents in the locality of ports were, therefore, put in jeopardy. As has been seen, even the migration of people from one locality, where the disease was rife, to another could cause a fresh outbreak. People usually kept themselves to themselves; strangers were, therefore, looked at suspiciously. Vagrants, sometimes called tramps, were rarely welcomed as they were also frequently responsible for spreading smallpox because of their itinerant way of life and their congregation in close proximity at night.

## Case history: Mary Barton, 1730

This woman provides a typical example of the attention that was thought necessary in 1730, and the resultant costs, for a pregnant vagrant with smallpox in the small parish of Bromham in north Bedfordshire, which is not known to have had a pesthouse.

*Bill for the charges of Mary Barton in Bromham, Bedfordshire, in 1730*

|  | £ | s | d |
|---|---|---|---|
| For 14 days board of the nurse nursing her and washing up the linen |  | 7 | 0 |
| For the vagrant's board and lodging and firing in her room |  | 7 | 6 |
| For soap and firing for washing the linen |  | 1 | 6 |
|  |  | 16 | 0 [£0.80] |

*Bill of charges of the constable of Bromham*

|  | £ | s | d |
|---|---|---|---|
| For 14 days hire of a nurse for the said Mary Barton |  | 13 | 0 |
| Paid midwife for laying her |  | 5 | 0 |
| For necessaries at her lying-in, and beer and sugar and other things with cordial |  | 10 | 0 |
| Her coffin |  | 8 | 0 |
| Parish dues |  | 2 | 6 |
| Affidavit |  | 1 | 0 |
| Hiring men for carrying her to the grave |  | 6 | 0 |
| Beer at the funeral |  | 4 | 0 |
| Paid two women for laying her out when dead |  | 2 | 0 |
|  | £2 | 11 | 6 [£2.58] |

*For a child of the said Mary Barton*

|  | £ | s | d |
|---|---|---|---|
| For a woman nursing the child for 14 days, and for eating | 1 | 0 | 0 |
| Paid a woman for laying out the child |  | 1 | 0 |
| Coffin |  | 4 | 0 |
| Parish dues |  | 2 | 6 |
| Affidavit |  | 1 | 0 |
|  | £1 | 8 | 6 [£1.43][33] |

Mary Barton and her infant received at least some nursing care due to an efficient parochial system; she was kept warm, fed and had her clothes washed. A midwife, probably with previous experience, delivered her, and a wet nurse fed the infant. When mother and child died, the parish paid for them to be laid out, for their coffins and other funeral expenses. The cost was borne by the local ratepayers. Technically, under the Act of Settlement, 1662, a stranger could be removed from the parish, if there was no prospect of work within 40 days. People in need were expected to return to their own parish where they were entitled to assistance from the overseers of the poor. Perhaps Mary Barton arrived too late in the village to be moved; certainly no necessary expense was spared on her behalf. The next case, a person with smallpox in Gloucestershire in 1816, shows how the amended 1662 Act was applied locally, and illustrates the variability of the parochial system. The case was, apparently, so controversial that it was reported in a distant newspaper, the *Cambridge Chronicle*, on 15 November 1816.

## Case history: Richard Godsall, 1816

This man had been working for a considerable time at Badgeworth in Gloucestershire, many miles from his home parish of Powick in Worcester-shire, when he was taken ill with confluent smallpox one Wednesday. The following Sunday, application was made on his behalf to the parish officers after divine service, who indicated that he should make his way back to his own home. Because he was so ill he could reach only Churchdown, about two miles away. He and his wife rested that night in a desolate barn without sustenance or extra clothing and struggled next day to reach the hamlet of Twigworth in the parish of St Mary de Lode, a journey of nearly three miles. As he was unable to proceed further he applied to the Overseer for relief, who had him put in a hay loft, where again he had no extra covers. In the morning the disease had made such rapid progress that 'he exhibited a sad spectacle of human misery, totally blind, and so weak and emaciated that he was unable to stand'. Nevertheless, the Overseer had him lifted into a cart and carried ten miles through intervening parishes until he reached Tewkesbury, where he was to be left. The only attention he received was from his wife, who supported him in her arms the whole way to save him from the jolting of the cart. In Tewkesbury, his wretched state apparently exceeded all description. He was immediately taken to the House of Industry, given the best medical aid and, 'every solacing effort ... but it was too late to save him and he languished in increasing affliction until Friday morning'. A coroner's inquest concluded that his death was greatly accelerated by his removal from Twigworth.[34]

In 1834, the Poor Law Amendment Act removed the main responsibility for care of sick paupers from individual parishes to more impersonal Boards of Guardians in large union workhouses. When they were first established, there was far more sick paupers than had been envisaged. Guardians built more sick wards, particularly for fevers, and were often obliged to take out contracts with other institutions to provide more space. The cramped conditions in the casual wards of these workhouses and in common lodging houses, established in the nineteenth century where vagrants (tramps), often slept, were frequently cited as the source of infection in Poor Law records. When this happened, all the occupants were put in quarantine. A tramp is believed to have introduced smallpox into the small market town of Ampthill, Bedfordshire, in 1882. The union workhouse was commandeered as a smallpox hospital and it provided some form of care for 150 of the most severe cases. Householders in afflicted premises were isolated in their own homes, but left a basket outside into which sympathisers could leave provisions. There were 19 deaths in this outbreak.[35]

It clearly caused the Board of Guardians concern: at their meeting on 2 February 1882, they noted that in consequence of a severe outbreak of smallpox at the workhouse, all communications with the workhouse had stopped because of the epidemic. Similar comments appeared in their fortnightly meetings until 13 April, when the term 'severe outbreak' was used for the last time. On 16 March a letter was read out from the LGB, concerned about the measures taken locally for vaccination and revaccination of the populace.[36] It is likely that only pauper nurses were available to attend the sick, although the Guardians had advertised earlier for a nurse at the workhouse. Apparently, only one application was received, from Eliza Lambes, 15 Bath Street, Hereford, but as no testimonials were sent it could not be considered at the meeting on 5 January. A letter requesting same was sent.[37] Throughout the eighteenth and nineteenth centuries, most people in Britain who contracted smallpox were isolated according to the availability of local resources. Their care was similarly haphazard.

Until the early 1890s it was still common practice to admit smallpox patients into general workhouse wards, despite being ordered to desist by the LGB. One such example was Dewsbury, Yorkshire.[38] Many voluntary hospitals discontinued this practice much earlier however, including Northampton General Hospital, the Bristol Infirmary and the London Hospital.[39] Few hospitals admitted patients with obvious signs of smallpox, although some cases became apparent only after admission as the disease was still in the incubation stage. In 1752, St Bartholomew's Hospital, London, decided to remove patients who had developed the disease to separate specialist wards.[40] In 1818, physicians at the Radcliffe Infirmary, Oxford, experienced difficulties with smallpox patients, although they were not supposed to be admitted as the Guardians of the Poor usually sent them to pesthouses.[41] As rural populations gradually declined, pesthouses fell into disuse and the wise eighteenth-century practice of isolation virtually fell into abeyance for much of the nineteenth century, except in some cities.

## Central government measures

The Sanitary Act, 1866, and the Public Health Act, 1875, authorised local authorities in England and Wales to establish fever (or isolation) hospitals, but relatively few conformed before the last decade of the nineteenth century. Although smallpox was usually more easily diagnosed than most infectious diseases, it was not possible to implement isolation and quarantine measures until a particular person had been identified, diagnosed and the existence of the disease made known to the local sanitary authority. It was not until the end of the nineteenth century that the Infectious Diseases Notification Act, 1889, made smallpox compulsorily notifiable in London and permissory elsewhere; the second such Act in 1899 made it compulsory throughout England and Wales.[42]

## The rise of smallpox hospitals

The first smallpox hospital in England was founded in London in 1746 at Cold Bath Fields, Clerkenwell, as a result of a charity created in 1740 to relieve poor persons suffering from smallpox. It was built on the site of a house previously used by the charity for the treatment of infected persons. The trustees had also owned land in St Pancras since 1765, when they had moved the Inoculation Hospital from a house in Old Street. In 1793–94, the hospital was rebuilt there and it then admitted patients from the Cold Bath Fields Hospital. As the land in St Pancras was being redeveloped as King's Cross Station (1850), the Smallpox Hospital moved to a site on Highgate Hill.[43] The rebuilt 100-bed London Smallpox Hospital was established in 1848–49 in extensive grounds on Highgate Hill. Although it was a voluntary hospital, many cases were sent, by arrangement, from workhouses and general hospitals; a governor's letter was required and fees were payable to cover the cost of the hospital stay.[44] As in outbreaks of fever, panic occurred in smallpox epidemics. The world-wide pandemic of 1870–73 was especially severe. In England, emergency hospitals were opened in many parts of the country,[45] but between epidemics, local authorities, particularly in inland rural areas, saw little need to finance rarely needed establishments.

In 1893, provincial county councils (but not county boroughs), were empowered to provide hospitals for infectious diseases, which included small-pox. The size and quality of such hospitals was very variable. The (Minority) Report of the Royal Commission on Poor Laws, 1905–09 (p. 876), noted that large areas of England still made do with 'the cottage or shed with two or three beds set aside for the occasional smallpox patient'.[46] Local authorities began to establish their own, or joint, smallpox hospitals, if they did not already exist. By 1914, there were 363 smallpox hospitals in England and Wales, in addition to fever, general, special hospitals and Poor Law infirmaries.[47] All vied with each other to attract nursing staff, but when there were epidemics, there was an even greater shortage of nurses. The smallpox hospitals varied considerably in size according to local need; for example, in 1922, Penro Smallpox Hospital, Aberystwyth, had just three beds, Little Bromwich, Birmingham, had 180, and the Robroyston Smallpox Hospital, Glasgow, had 448 beds.[48] Small hospitals were often empty for years and thus were not in a state of readiness when need arose, but larger ones were more likely to be kept busy, particularly in port areas. As a result of the LGB view that smallpox could be transmitted by 'aerial convection', the Board insisted that smallpox hospitals should not be sited within half a mile of a population of 600 persons. In order to obtain loans to establish new hospitals, local authorities had to adhere to these conditions, laid down in 1902.[49]

## The situation in London

Infectious disease, be it endemic, epidemic, or even pandemic,[50] is a powerful motivator towards action to protect the well from the sick. The larger the city, the more visible the problem. London was, for centuries, hugely bigger than any other city. It became pre-eminent in Britain and in Europe by the end of the seventeenth century. Between 1600 and 1700 the population is believed to have risen from 200,000 to 575,000 persons, and by 1800 to 900,000 persons, 10 per cent of the total English population. Such density, often with cramped living conditions, encouraged crowd diseases such as smallpox and measles.[51]

The endemic nature of smallpox in the capital came to the attention of the Registrar General for England and Wales following the introduction of the compulsory civil registration of births and deaths from 1837, which replaced the unreliable parish registration system. In 1841, William Farr (1807–83), Statistical Superintendent in the Registrar General's Office (1838–80), a pioneer in the application of 'vital statistics' in England and Wales, wrote poignantly about children in London who were unprotected by vaccination. At least five were destroyed daily; they did not die suddenly with little pain, but lingered many days before they perished. Survivors, he wrote, escaped as if from the fire with cicatrised (scarred) faces, irreparably deformed and 'perhaps blinded for life'.[52] In fact, smallpox was rarely absent from London in the years leading to 1900.[53] This was one of the reasons a new system was introduced.

In 1867, a central authority for infectious diseases (and insanity), namely, the Metropolitan Asylums Board (MAB), was established.[54] It stamped out smallpox in the capital, firstly by the establishment of the land ambulance service in 1881, and secondly, by the inauguration of the river service in 1884, which avoided taking patients through London and enabled patients to be transported in paddle steamers to the marquees set up to form the 300 bed South Smallpox Camp at Darenth, Kent. The hospital tents each contained 20 beds which rested on wooden floors. The Board also established river hospitals at Dartford in Kent in 1902. Initially, however, it used temporary establishments including the Hampstead Smallpox Hospital (1870), and the quarantine hulk, *Dreadnought*, moored at Greenwich in the epidemic of 1871–72. Two other hulks served the same purpose in the epidemic of 1880–81. They were moved in 1882 to the south bank of the River Thames at Long Reach, Dartford, where the MAB had purchased land.[55]

Isla Stewart (later Matron, St Bartholomew's Hospital, London, 1887–1910) was appointed Matron of this camp during the 1884–85 epidemic. The separate male and female camps comprised 22 tents for patients, one for the Matron, and others for general purposes and for the staff. The Medical Superintendent lived in a house previously used as the farmhouse.[56] Miss Stewart described the appalling conditions which had to be endured at the tented hospital in wet weather, when chalk from the hillside made the floors cold, wet and slippery. The hot pipes made the air inside the tents stuffy, and in winter, when everyone was crowded together, the extreme offensiveness of the disease was unavoidable, as was the never to be forgotten penetrating odour. A nursing staff of several hundred cared for the 1,800 patients, 'mostly under canvas'. In 1888 she explained that doctors believed that smallpox was a 'nurses' disease'.[57] As with other potentially fatal infectious diseases, when cure was not possible, care was, predominantly, the nurses' prerogative.

## Smallpox: a nurses' disease

The term 'nurses' disease' can be interpreted as a general acknowledgement of the importance of good nursing care, although recovery was also dependent on other factors, such as the patient's age, constitution and the virulence of the disease. When the standard of care was good, the patient had a better chance of recovery, perhaps with less disfigurement, provided that the rash was properly treated. Even when the patient's death was inevitable, the last days could be made more comfortable. Moreover, the nurse who carried out necessary duties with strict attention to isolation techniques, even after death (when the body was still contagious), could prevent the spread of the disease, not only to others, but also to herself. In the last major British outbreak in 1902, of the 7,916 patients admitted to the smallpox hospitals managed by the MAB, 1,337 died, a 17 per cent mortality rate.[58] It is likely to have been much higher were it not for the provision of efficient nursing care. The MAB employed male nurses for the first time in this epidemic.[59]

The other interpretation of the term 'nurses' disease' is one which recognises that nurses could contract the disease themselves as a result of their work. Some did so, unwittingly, in hospitals, asylums and workhouse infirmaries during the nineteenth and early twentieth centuries, either because the disease had not become manifest when patients were admitted in the incubation stage, or strict segregation of infectious diseases was not always followed. Misdiagnosis could put nurses further at risk. For example, in the decennial period 1894–1903 the percentage of misdiagnosis of smallpox cases examined at the South Wharf before admission to the MAB hospital ships at Dartford ranged from 7.7– 83.3 per cent.[60] Staff who worked in any institution, whatever their role, were at risk of contracting the disease, but nurses, because of their necessarily close contact with patients, bore the greatest risk.

A LGB report (1880–81) contains a statement that nurses in early times were 'selected from among those who had passed through an attack of small-pox' and latterly 'having their vaccination specially cared for, took nothing from their patients'.[61] Nevertheless, some nurses, and others working with patients, usually because they were unprotected by effective vaccination, did contract smallpox and some died from its effects. However, they probably had scant awareness of the risk they were taking: it failed to prevent many from volunteering, heroically, for duty, mostly because they had never met the awful reality of this loathsome disease. This issue is not clear cut as examples have been found in England and abroad, where nurses were compelled to nurse smallpox patients. In a very severe epidemic of smallpox in the Cape Peninsula, South Africa, in 1812, public health measures included vaccination, quarantine regulations and the setting up of emergency hospitals. At the acute hospital established on Paarden Island, the death rate was 48.8 per cent, indicating the particularly virulent nature of the disease. Slaves who had had smallpox and were, therefore, immune, were used as nurses in the hospital and in patients' own homes where they could be isolated. Some of the attendants were 'Free Blacks, and a few of the women attendants were "Cape Coloured" '.[62] Over a century later, at the 46-bedded Infectious Hospital, Friarton, Perth in Scotland, the rules (1919) for nurses stated that, 'In the event of Smallpox breaking out in the City or neighbourhood, to submit to re-vaccination (if not already done), and to undertake the nursing of Smallpox when required'.[63]

Many instances of courageous devotion to duty have been found, but only a few are cited here. During an epidemic at Three Counties Asylum, Bedfordshire, in 1884–85 (56 cases, with 14 deaths), an extra hospital build-ing was 'staffed entirely by volunteers', of whom two contracted the disease and one died.[64] The records of the London Smallpox Hospital, Highgate, indicate that some surgeons, medical attendants and medical students contracted the disease. Nurses from the London Hospital in Whitechapel, one of the poorest areas of the capital, were particularly vulnerable. Although two probationers contracted smallpox, Catherine Hore, aged 28 years in 1883, and Margaret Miller, aged 23 years in 1884, both recovered. The Royal Free Hospital paid five guineas (£5.25) for the care of their nurse, Elizabeth McHarter, aged 31 years, admitted 29 May 1885 with 'pustular malignant with pneumonia', who died on 4 June 1885. Her vaccination marks showed only 'two poor cicatrices'.[65]

MAB records also provide evidence of nurses who contracted smallpox, either in its own hospitals or elsewhere. During the 1902 epidemic in London, Dr Ricketts, the Medical Superintendent of the smallpox ships and hospitals at Dartford, was obliged to accept unvaccinated nurses to work there, 'on the understanding that they would be vaccinated immediately on arrival'. Even recent vaccination failed to confer immunity at times, although it offered some protection. Assistant Nurse Gregory, who had been revaccinated at the Northern Hospital, Winchmore Hill, was transferred on

15 March 1902 to the Long Reach Hospital where, including the hospital ships, there were 320 smallpox patients. On 4 April, she contracted a very mild form of the disease. In 1922, there were 69 notifications of smallpox in the London boroughs, 51 of which were in Poplar; 16 of these died.[66] One of these was Nurse E.C.C., aged 24 years, who 'should have been protected by revaccination' at the Poplar Institution, but who died at the Long Reach Hospital in November 1922.[67]

In the Edinburgh outbreak (1942), all the fever nursing staff of the City Hospital, Edinburgh, volunteered, despite the 'prolonged restrictions and privations'. Two senior sisters and the eleven 'most reliable senior probationers' were selected, plus two female volunteers from the wartime Casualty Services, none of whom succumbed to the disease. By then, the risk of recently revaccinated nurses contracting smallpox was thought to be negligible.[68] Nevertheless, some nurses still died. An outbreak in Glasgow (1950) was believed to have originated from an Asian seaman, Mussa Ali, from the liner *Chitral*, which docked at Tilbury on 5 March. He, apparently, took the disease to Glasgow and was admitted to the Knightswood Fever Hospital, before being transferred to Robroyston Hospital where, by 28 March, he was said to be recovering.[69] Nevertheless, on 11 April that year, Catherine Wilson (20), who had nursed him at Knightswood, died from smallpox. Two other nurses and a laundry worker from this hospital were 'earlier victims of the disease'.[70]

Isla Stewart's account of the nursing care (outlined earlier with regard to the situation in London) carried out during the 1884–85 epidemic in London, in which MAB organised accommodation for patients in hospital ships and tents, probably provides the most illuminating insight of how a professionally trained nurse managed the situation, although she found it difficult because the 'greatest blot' was the nursing. Few nurses were trained; the work was carried out by mostly 'excellent women', but who lacked knowledge. For confluent cases, Miss Stewart advocated an airy environment, kept at a uniform temperature. Although the delirium could be violent, as little restraint as possible should be used, while constantly keeping the patient under observation. Tepid sponging could relieve a high temperature. The eyes should be carefully watched and kept clean; any soreness or swelling should be drawn to the doctor's attention immediately. Vaseline might relieve irritation. A water bed should be used for the patient and the mouth kept as clean as possible. As haematuria (blood in the urine) is a grave sign, the urine should be observed and the bowels should be kept open. In cases of confluent smallpox, soreness usually prevents combing, which leads to pediculi congregating and multiplying under the scabs. The hair should, therefore, be cut off as closely as possible and carbolic oil applied. To 'facilitate scabing' [*sic*], a piece of lint can be cut into the shape of the face with holes for the eyes, nose and mouth, then smeared with vaseline before applying it to the face. In discrete cases little care is necessary, but in those with the haemorrhagic form, there is little to do, 'except to soothe the last days of the unfortunate patient'.[71]

Among the comprehensive records kept by medical and nursing staff on the MAB hospital ships *Atlas*, *Endymion* and *Castalia*, moored at Long Reach, in the Thames Estuary, is the case history of Elizabeth Slade (Figures 5.2 and 5.3).

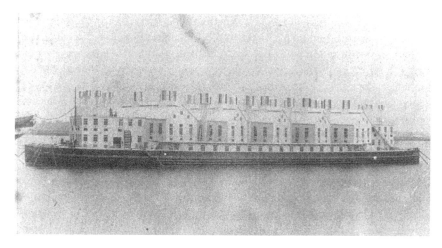

*Figure 5.2* Hospital ship, *Castalia*, showing wards in echelon, Long Reach, Dartford, Kent, 1884–1904. London Metropolitan Archives

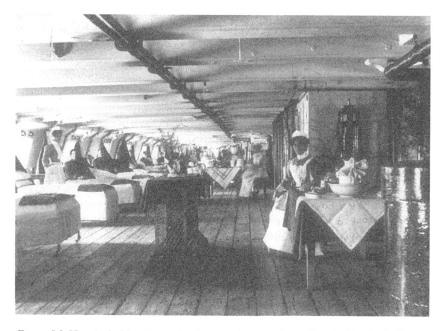

*Figure 5.3* Hospital ship, *Atlas*, showing ward scene, Long Reach, Dartford, Kent, 1881–1904. London Metropolitan Archives

## Case history: Elizabeth Slade, 1894

Elizabeth Slade, aged 23 years, lived with her mother and father, a florist, at 56 Richmond Street, Lisson Grove, Marylebone, London. On 4 December 1894, she became ill and vomited. On 7 December, a rash erupted on her hands and she was admitted to the MAB South Western Fever Hospital, Stockwell. She was transferred to the floating hospital ship *Castalia*, and admitted to ward C4 on 8 December, under the care of Dr T. F. Ricketts, the Medical Superintendent. A diagnosis of confluent smallpox was made. Elizabeth had a profuse papular rash, but none on the palms of her hands. She had not been vaccinated, but had apparently had smallpox at 3 years of age. Her religion is given as Church of England. It was learned that a case of smallpox had been removed from the same street on 5 December.

Her medical case notes, which are very detailed, written over the next few days show that she was seen by a doctor at least once daily. She was prescribed a 'Sick ii' diet, which included beef tea and bread and milk, plus a number of extras: bottles of soda water, new-laid eggs, oranges, milk, port wine and brandy. A wide range of medication was prescribed, for example, sulphonal (a hypnotic) and paraldehyde (a soporific) and a glycerine solution for her mouth, which was clearly dry and uncomfortable. Poultices to throat and ice compresses to eyes and forehead, fomentations to neck, tepid and cold sponging were also ordered, and carried out by the nurses. On the day of admission, the rash was fairly profuse and 'deeply' papular over her left forearm and left leg from the knee, but still vesicular in a few places. There were also signs of a small confluent patch, almost exactly similar in distribution and extent to that on her right side. The rash was done up 'Aseptically' at 8 p.m., which clearly made Elizabeth more comfortable, as on 12 December she asked to have her right side done up in the same way. On 13 December, the rash became fully pustular; her hands and feet, especially below the bandage, were very swollen. She was sick twice during the day.

The doctor continued to monitor and record changes in her rash and general condition, and order whatever was necessary. On 16 December it was decided that she should not have any solid food, that is, bread and milk; she was to have an enema if her bowels were not open, her hair was to be cut close and her arms were no longer to be wrapped in mackintosh. However, damp cloths could be used if necessary. On 17 December, her throat, which had caused her pain previously, revealed a sloughing deep ulcer and a special mixture was prescribed with which to paint it. Her pulse was 140 beats per minute; there was less oedema of her extremities, and the rash was drying up in many places on her arms and legs. The pocks were now not nearly so tense anywhere.

The nurses' reports, written by day and night staff, show how closely Elizabeth was observed and the attention she received. They include twice daily and four hourly temperature charts, recorded in the Fahrenheit (F) scale, which show a continued fever, that is, it did not return to a normal level (98.4°F or 37°C) (Figure 5.4). During her illness, her temperature ranged

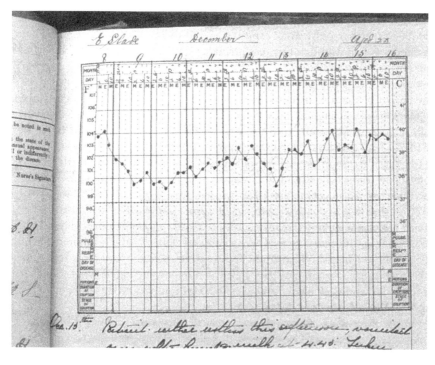

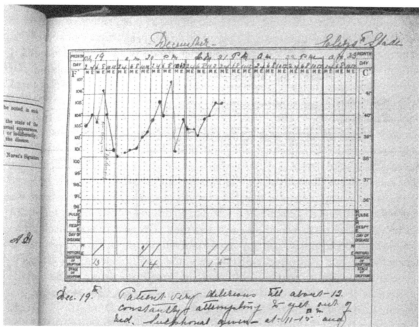

*Figure 5.4* Temperature charts, Elizabeth Slade, 1894. Jenner Museum, Berkeley, Gloucestershire

from 99.6 to 106.8°F on 20 December, at 8 p.m. The nurses, apparently, did not document her pulse and respirations, but did record her motions. They ensured she had as much food and drink as she could manage and reported any adverse signs, such as her cough and difficulty with breathing and the amount of sleep she had. Most nights, and some days, she was very restless. She had little sleep. During the early hours of 12 December, she complained of 'Choking' and coughed more frequently. Medicine was given and she slept from 2.30 a.m. to 5 a.m., but not afterwards. She was inclined to be 'light headed'. The poultices, which were applied two hourly, gave her relief.

Elizabeth's condition slowly declined. She became very restless and vomited at times. The brandy was usually accepted well, but on 15 December she objected 'to it very much'. Her temperature was reduced from 104 to 102.2°F that day by tepid sponging for ten minutes. During most of her illness she drank copious quantities of milk and took some of the extras. On 16 December she was very drowsy all day and slept for about an hour in the afternoon; her breathing was laboured between 2 and 4 p.m.; her temperature was 105°F. An enema was given – her bowels 'acted well'. She felt comfortable and slept after being washed. Her temperature at the end of the day was 102.8°F; she had not vomited.

On 19 December, Elizabeth was very delirious until about 12 midday, 'constantly attempting to get out of bed'. Sulphonal was given at 11.15 a.m. and repeated one hour later. She slept from 12.30 to 1.20 p.m., suddenly gave a deep sigh and had twitching of her face and arm, left side; the right arm was very slightly affected. The twitching occurred again at 2.25 p.m., but was much worse and lasted for about four minutes. 'Patient does not speak when spoken to – but seems to understand all that is said to her. Ice bag to head'. On 20 December, her condition deteriorated; her speech, which had returned, was rambling, she was very delirious and in a comatose condition from 3.35 p.m. She was tepid sponged for ten minutes, but her temperature was still recorded at 104°F. The medical notes, however, show that her temperature was 106.8°F and that she was quite comatose with a very feeble pulse. She was given a cold bath at 8.30 p.m. after which 'she was very cold and pulse bad and had hot bottle, and blankets for about 10 mins'. After the bath, although 'rather collapsed', she was conscious and able to swallow and had about half an ounce of brandy in three hours. As she was able to take so little by mouth, she was given a nutrient enema comprising one ounce each of beef tea, milk and brandy, which she retained, but was unable to retain a second one next morning. The twitchings continued on both sides of her face; she still appeared conscious at times. Her condition was clearly failing, but the doctor, aided by the nurses, still made valiant efforts to save her life; despite further cold sponging, her temperature could not be reduced. At 12 midday it was 105°F with a very rapid pulse, 'almost imperceptible'. She died at 2.35 p.m. on 21 December.[72]

It is clear from this case history that the care and treatment ordered was of a high standard. Every change was monitored and a nurse was in constant attention. Elizabeth's illness appears to have been so serious that recovery was not possible. She was one of the 89 people in London who died of the disease that year, when there was a mortality rate of 22 per million persons due to smallpox. The previous year, 1893, there were 206 deaths with a mortality rate of 48 per million persons.[73]

## Management of outbreaks

London, and a few other large cities, were exceptional in providing enough hospital accommodation; be it in tents, ships or buildings, nurses were expected to adapt to the situation. In the late nineteenth century, some smallpox patients were still nursed at home where the local Medical Officer of Health, was responsible for organising nursing care. In 1893, Horace Sworder, part-time MOH for the Urban District of Luton, published a small book with information about smallpox. He advised that if the patient could not be removed to a fever hospital, everyone in the house should be vaccinated or revaccinated, unless this had recently been carried out or if a very young child had good vaccination marks. A good nurse must be secured, but better still, two nurses in case of delirium as the patient should never be left. As the scabs are so highly infectious, they should be treated with carbolic oil and, when they fall off, burnt. Finally, disinfection must always be carried out under the superintendence of the Inspector of Nuisances.[74] In private houses, and particularly in small hospitals, it was not unusual for nurses to lift the still contagious body into the coffin before interment.

An ideal nurse in an epidemic would be one who had had the disease or been vaccinated and recently revaccinated, with knowledge and practical experience gained in previous epidemics. Ability to understand different languages would be useful, especially in port areas. A cheerful, resilient personality would facilitate mixing with patients and staff, enable the nurse to withstand the revulsion caused by the distressing sight and unpleasant smell associated with more serious forms of the disease, and cope with the harrowing death of patients, and sometimes colleagues. However, relatively few fever nurses in the twentieth century encountered smallpox patients. As hardly any available nurses were likely to have had all the above attributes, patients were often cared for by anyone suitable in epidemics, including what were then termed 'co-op' or agency nurses.

Before the advent of fever nurse training, there was usually one competent general trained nurse who insisted that strict régimes of care, including proper isolation techniques, were followed in epidemics. This authoritarian approach usually resulted in praise following the crisis. Documentary evidence provides examples of such women capable of taking command in a crisis. As discussed previously, Miss Stewart managed the smallpox camps at Darenth in 1884–85, when there were 1,800 patients and 'several hundred male and female nurses'. She 'reduced the chaos she found to some sort of order.' When the camp was closed, a special record was made of her services and faithful discharge of her duties.[75] Likewise, in the 1897–98 Middlesbrough outbreak, Miss Bell, Matron of the local sanatorium, organised care for 1,405 patients, 201 of whom died, a very low mortality rate of 14 per cent. In an account of the epidemic, published by the local newspaper, Miss Bell was extolled for managing affairs 'with an almost military manner, so strict is the discipline at the Hospital'.[76] Discipline applied to many areas of nursing practice. For instance, nursing staff and others in quarantine during an outbreak of smallpox were expressly forbidden to leave the premises and mix with other people. Smallpox was believed to be spread, not just by droplet infection to close contacts and clothing, but by the airborne route. Consequently, illicit contact by staff with people outside the hospital was often cited as a possible source of the spread of the disease, as were flies.[77]

## Smallpox outbreak in a Poor Law Infirmary, c.1901–02

The best example found of a trained nurse and midwife who coped with a smallpox outbreak in appalling circumstances in the first years of the twentieth century was published some years later in the *Nursing Times* in 1926. She was careful not to reveal her name or any other identifiable details, but there is sufficient evidence to date it.

She had trained in a London Poor Law infirmary with over 600 beds, with three months spent in medical, surgical, mental and maternity wards and had lectures given by the medical men. She was one of the first nurses to gain the London Obstetric Society certificate, the first examination for which was held in 1872.[78] This nurse later accepted a position as charge nurse in a country Poor Law infirmary where the master had been in post for 40 years and his daughter acted as Matron. The doctor, also elderly, lived a mile away and was not often called. In this situation, smallpox broke out in 1901–02. A section of this article is quoted verbatim as it reveals, in her own words, the sheer horror of the appalling circumstances in which she was expected to work; it also reveals her efficiency and attention to detail.

> One morning the master came over to me and said he was sending over a man from the tramp ward who had been admitted the night before and had a rash, but had been allowed to mix with the other people. The master thought a little mild ointment would cure the rash, but during the night the man had become delirious, and when he was sent to me I found he had a temperature ranging from 104 upwards. I refused to do anything till the doctor was sent for, and when he came he found as I had suspected a very bad case of smallpox. He had the man removed to a little isolation ward, a very rough place, at the back of the infirmary, with one of my feeble-minded helpers to look after him. The thing spread like wildfire, till in addition to my usual patients I had 38 cases of smallpox. No nurse could be got for a time, for smallpox was raging all over England just then, so after I had done the general patients I used to undress in an out-house, put on an overall I kept there, and do what I could for the suffering smallpox

patients, finding one morning one of my best helpers lying dead on the floor in a pool of blood [haemorrhagic smallpox], to my grief and horror. Before going back to the infirmary I used to get into a bath with a strong disinfectant in it, and in that way purify myself as far as possible before going near the general patients. To add to my anxiety I had three lying-in patients, and I was in constant terror lest they should be infected. I spoke to the doctor about it, and he said smallpox was not so injurious to lying-in patients as scarlet fever, and spoke rather as if it might be actually helpful to them than otherwise! However, thank God they all escaped, and we stopped at 38 cases, eight of whom died. I rolled the bodies in sheets saturated with carbolic, then measured them for their coffins, sent the measurements to the undertaker, and his men brought the coffins and put them through the hedge at the bottom of the garden, while I and my men helpers fetched them, put the bodies in and screwed them down, with prayer on our lips and in our hearts for those who had gone and those of us who remained. We wondered who would be the next, but there was too much to do and we had no time to worry about ourselves.

Part of my infirmary was set aside for the smallpox cases, and we had three tents in the grounds; it was in June, and very hot weather; no one was allowed out from the infirmary for nine weeks, but I often spent the whole night in the grounds, getting what sleep I could in a hammock. How I lived through that time I don't know. At last a nurse was got for the smallpox cases, but as she told the authorities an untruth and said she had been vaccinated when she hadn't, she had not been long on duty before she, too, developed smallpox and was very ill. Someone else had to be got to look after them, and till we could get them I had to go on as I did before. However it came to an end at last.[79]

It could be argued that the master and doctor involved at this workhouse were ineffective as they were unused to coping with an epidemic on this scale. Nevertheless, it resulted in a mortality rate of only 21 per cent, probably due to the strict isolation measures the nurse observed, which prevented more inmates contracting the disease, and the long nine-week period of quarantine, which prevented its spread into the wider community. The issue of vaccination was very relevant to this nurse and to others in similar epidemics. Compulsory vaccination had been in force in some parts of Europe since the early nineteenth century: Bavaria (1807), Denmark (1810), Hesse and other German states and effectively Prussia (1818), causing a dramatic fall in mortality rates from smallpox.[80] A 'Report as to Smallpox Accommodation' in Edinburgh, dated 17 October 1910, observed that except for the town of Mainz, separate smallpox hospitals were not required in the German Empire as vaccination and revaccination were enforced. As the population was 'perfectly protected by their vaccination and revaccination, at school age and military service age', it was thought safe to treat smallpox patients in general hospitals.[81] In Britain, people railed against enforcement.

The Vaccination Act, 1853, had made the vaccination of infants compulsory within three months of birth, but this Act was not effective. From 1871, parents who refused to have their child vaccinated were likely to be fined or imprisoned. Under the 'conscience clause' in the Vaccination Act, 1898, parents could opt out of vaccination legally. It is clear from the literature that this measure frustrated local MOHs, trying to prevent the spread of the disease. The general opinion of the medical profession in 1902 was that smallpox hospitals and the large expenditure entailed in dealing with small-pox outbreaks would be entirely unnecessary if effective vaccination and revaccination were made compulsory. 'Certainly all tramps ought to be periodically vaccinated, for the majority of small-pox outbreaks are caused by vagrants disseminating the disease'.[82]

## Poorly vaccinated communities

An unvaccinated population meant that there were potentially more patients requiring nursing care following an outbreak of smallpox. It also signified a threat to the local economy. Luton was one of a number of towns which had a poor record for vaccination. For instance, in 1909, the first full year of school medical inspection in the Borough, of 2,205 children inspected, only 211 had been vaccinated – a very low 9.5 per cent.[83] In 1909, the New Industries Committee was succeeding in attracting new labour to the town, particularly men needed in the engineering works and, to a lesser extent, the hat trade. Some workers initially availed themselves of sleeping quarters in common lodging houses. There were four such licensed houses in the borough with a total of 25 rooms, 112 beds and (apparently) accommodation for 132 persons per night. In 1909, 41,073 persons used these facilities, an increase of 15,932 persons in the previous year.[84] Purpose-built casual wards were opened in 1904 at Luton Union Workhouse, to provide accommodation for vagrants and, if necessary, their families. These wards, situated in what resembled a stable block, could accommodate up to 100 men, women and children, every week, as they were required to move to another town after two nights. An extension to the casual wards was opened in 1927 and by 1929 as many as 500 persons were accommodated every week.[85] Demographic change is known to exacerbate the spread of infection.

In the late 1920s and 1930s, many areas in Britain were in economic decline. Workers flooded into Luton from the depressed areas of Tyneside, Clydeside and South Wales to take up work in the hat trade and the various engineering works including Vauxhall Motors, Skefko, Commer Cars, Kents and Electrolux. On 5 March 1928, a casual at the Luton Union Workhouse, who may have been seeking employment, was discovered to be infected with smallpox; he was, therefore, removed to be isolated at Codicote.[86] According to Mrs Margaret Bracey (previously Sister (Ivy) Sheldon) in 1982, who was Sister-in-charge of the Infirmary in 1928, 'all the nurses had to be vaccinated and then isolated within the confines of the walls'.[87] This one case, therefore, had considerable consequences for other patients and nurses. On 31 May, a further case was discovered in Gaitskill Terrace, Luton, a known socially deprived area. Neither he, nor the other thirteen cases had been vaccinated. As a result of one of these cases, a Bedford contact who worked in a large hat factory in Luton, a hundred contacts were vaccinated. The Sanitary Committee of Luton Borough Council recorded their appreciation of the efficient manner in which the MOH, William Archibald, and his staff (which included health visitors and hospital nurses), dealt with the outbreak.[88]

There were no notifications of smallpox in Luton in the years 1929–31, but the disease broke out again in 1932. From 8 February to 8 June, there were forty-nine cases, all unvaccinated except for five who had been vaccinated in infancy. All were, apparently, treated in the Borough Smallpox Hospital with a staff of two nurses and one maid. The MOH reported that about 400 extra hours were put in by the Sanitary Inspector and the Senior Health Visitor, without whose work, he believed, there was no 'knowing to what extent the epidemic might have spread and the effect it would have had on the town's industries'. Under the Public Health (Smallpox Prevention) Regulations, 1917, as many as 2,040 vaccinations or revaccinations were carried out in factories, which enabled employees from all areas of the town and surrounding villages to be dealt with 'on the spot'.[89] The practically unvaccinated state of the community, which may well have included some recent migrant groups to the town, meant extra work for the Sanitary Department and the Smallpox Hospital. Certainly, two nurses and a maid seem to have been rather inadequate for twenty-four-hour cover for the four months' duration of this epidemic at the hospital. However, Luton was by no means the only place which had a poorly protected community.

Grimsby, in Lincolnshire, had a 70 per cent unvaccinated population, when an outbreak of variola major occurred on 17 February 1947; there were fifteen cases, all male, six of whom died, a 40 per cent mortality rate, probably because of the severity of the disease. Nevertheless, Miss E. D. MacKenzie, Matron, Grimsby Corporation Hospital, who took charge in terrible winter conditions, was applauded for her work. The local MOH, James A. Kerr, paid tribute to her and others, who despite the arctic weather 'exhibited a spirit of keenness and teamwork'. Miss Mackenzie, 'by reason of her experience in hospital administration and her power of leadership, was a tower of strength'. The disease was provisionally diagnosed by a senior nurse with recent experience of smallpox in North Africa. Due to deep snow, the road to Grimsby Smallpox Hospital at Laceby, could not be opened for forty-eight hours; the first patient was, therefore, admitted to an ordinary empty ward at the local isolation hospital. Enough nursing and domestic staff, who had been vaccinated within the previous twelve months, volunteered to live, sleep and eat on the ward.[90]

The patient, a male aged 75 years, lived in a common lodging house with about twenty-four other permanent inmates. Although he had not been out for about six weeks due to the severe weather, new inmates from 'a minority of floating population' there caused tremendous problems with contact tracing because of poor record keeping. Three persons had been admitted to Scartho Road Infirmary from the lodging house, one of whom, an unvaccinated man of 85 years, had died of pneumonia. Examination of the body post-mortem showed the smallpox rash in the very early stages and new lesions which had appeared since death. Unfortunately, nine nurses at the infirmary had never been vaccinated. Primary vaccination was immediately carried out, 'which shook them considerably'. They then gave blood so that the serum would be available for other cases. Penicillin had no effect on the original smallpox infection, but it had a marked effect on the secondary infection and greatly reduced scarring. The relatively new drug was given in a dosage of 30,000 units, three hourly in serious cases and 100,000 units in oil three times daily in less serious cases. It was thought most desirable to commence this treatment at least forty-eight hours before there was likely to be any pyrexia due to secondary sepsis. One case who had not had penicillin early enough needed his sheets changing twice every day because of the 'pouring out of pus'.[91] It is evident that nurses at all levels were needed but fever nurse probationers probably carried out most patient care.[92] They were the most economical and malleable workforce, but, as was seen in Chapter 2, it was seldom found easy to recruit and retain them. The best strategy was to offer a contract of training.

## Smallpox training

Smallpox nursing was never a separate registerable qualification; it was an integral part of fever nurse training. However, it had not begun on a national scale by the time of the last major smallpox epidemic in 1901–02. Mr A. C. Sewell, chairman of the MAB Hospitals Committee in London, showed his dismay and regret that during the epidemic, the supply of trained nurses was less than the demand, a disgrace, 'a decided reflection on the nursing profession as a whole'.[93] As was seen in Chapter 2, some large isolation hospitals had begun fever training in the late nineteenth century. In 1909, the Fever Nurses' Association drafted a syllabus of eight lectures on anatomy and physiology, and twelve lectures on fevers and fever nursing. This was approved by the MAB for use in its fever hospitals and was published in 1909. Smallpox was covered in Lecture X, which required the following topics to be taught: causation; symptoms; complications; modes of death; what to observe and report; preventive measures: vaccination and clinical nursing.[94] Other hospitals, approved by the FNA, adopted this syllabus. The *British Journal of Nursing* carried typical examination questions for the certificate of fever training. In April 1914, the paper included a question on the isolation and nursing of an infectious case in a private house and one on the infectious material associated with smallpox.[95] As mentioned in Chapter 3, the curriculum for fever nurses pioneered by the FNA in 1909 was adopted virtually unchanged by the three new General Nursing Councils after the

Registration Acts, 1919. Moreover, for the first time, the subjects of infectious diseases and the nature and spread of bacterial and surgical infections were laid down for all probationers undertaking an approved course in general nursing in Britain.[96]

Following the decline of variola major in Britain after 1902, fewer doctors and nurses became capable of differentiating between a severe case of chickenpox and one of variola minor. Emphasis on this problem in training and relevant examination questions ensured the issue was not forgotten. The Final State Examination in Fevers and Fever Nursing in England and Wales, in October 1938, included this compulsory question. 'Describe the symptoms which usually precede the characteristic eruption of Small-pox. State the main differences usually found between the eruptions of Small-pox and Chicken-pox'.[97] Once the various courses became established, there was a need for more theoretical knowledge. Although Matrons or Sister Tutors usually gave nursing care lectures, the medical staff were mainly responsible for enlightening probationers about diseases. It is possible to glean further information about smallpox nursing in the twentieth century from textbooks. Dr F. J. Woolacott reminded nurses in 1906 that it was not their duty to originate treatment, but it was sometimes very convenient, 'when she is sufficiently well-informed to anticipate and prepare for the instructions that are likely to be given her'. He mentioned that a male attendant may be necessary as, on occasions, the delirium assumes a violent form, and he warned that the disease could still be transmitted from the body of the patient after death, and by means of clothing or other articles.[98]

In *c.*1914, Miss Riddell, an experienced general nurse and lecturer, emphasised the need for skilful nursing. It encompassed many aspects of care, including frequent changing of bedlinen and clothing, absolute isolation and an emollient such as vaseline or oil of eucalyptus to allay skin irritation and to loosen the scabs. Warm baths might be given if the patient's condition permits and iced compresses 'applied to the face if there is much pain and swelling'. To relieve the severe itching she advocated sponging the body with dilute acetic acid and water. The eyes, which required special care, should be bathed frequently with boracic lotion and a weak solution of perchloride of mercury to keep them clean. Like her medical counterpart, she felt that a male attendant should be used when there was delirium. She reminded nurses that the infection, which had a very disagreeable odour, lasted from incubation until all discharges and desquamation (removal of epidermis by scaling) had ceased. This might be for eight to ten weeks.[99] Thus nurses, like their patients, would have been socially isolated.

In 1939, Joyce Watson, a sister tutor in fever nursing, wisely included protective measures for the nurse, as well as care of the patient, from leaving home (following which the dwelling, bedding and clothing had to be rigorously disinfected), until the patient recovered or died. Nurses, when on smallpox duty, were required to submit to strict quarantine, wear hooded linen overalls over their uniform (sometimes called 'wrappers') and use overshoes. They should take particular care of their general health and their hands; in severe cases, rubber gloves were to be worn. On leaving the hospital, they had to undergo thorough personal disinfection. Floors had to be mopped and damp dusting carried out with Izal; old sheets were recommended, which could then be burned. Otherwise linen should be soaked in a coal-tar disinfectant for two hours before laundering. An open fire was thought desirable to destroy all swabs soiled with discharges. Nurses were informed that urine, faeces and washing water also had to be disinfected before disposal.[100]

As the patient began to recover, 'a generous diet' was indicated to help prevent late complications including boils and abscesses. A meat diet was advocated with plenty of vegetables, fruit, eggs and cheese; adults might be allowed stout. Miss Watson also gave useful nursing 'tips' about how to deal with the highly infectious scabs on the soles of the feet, termed 'seeds'. They could be cut away using special fine curved scissors once the inflammation around them had subsided. Patients could not be discharged until all lesions were healed and the scabs separated, which could take from three weeks to three months. Nurses were warned that great care was necessary when dealing with a dead body. It was usual to wrap it completely in a carbolic soaked sheet and inter it in the hospital cemetery. The undertaker, who must have been vaccinated, should bath and disinfect himself after coffining the body.[101] The fine detail in this book was almost certainly of great value for nurses who seldom met patients with this disease. Those nursing in port areas were more likely to see the disease than those inland. The pattern of smallpox being repeatedly introduced at sea ports has often caused comment. In the seven-year period 1911–17, a total of 842 cases of smallpox were notified in Britain, 238 of which were in port towns and 101 in port sanitary districts, a percentage rate of 40 per cent.[102]

## Evidence from smallpox nurses

Oral and written evidence from nurses questioned in the 1997–98 study of fever nursing help to illuminate the reality of smallpox nursing and reinforce other research. Lists of nurses who had volunteered to nurse these patients were usually kept in Matron's Office. There was a sense of disappointment if one was not required, for example, 'we were once put on alert, but the expected outbreak did not occur' and 'the patient died before it was my turn'. When an outbreak occurred, it was usually senior probationers who were called. They knew that they had to remain in quarantine until there was no longer any chance of the disease spreading, but they were consoled by the fact that they often earned double pay, sometimes a bonus and additional leave.[103] Fever nurses based near ports were more likely to nurse smallpox patients, who were usually seamen, but sometimes foreign visitors, who often did not speak English. Very ill patients were admitted from ports in Liverpool (1935–38), Swansea (1937–41), London (Dartford, 1939–42) and

Bristol (1945–46). During 1934–36, a fever nurse probationer nursed small-pox patients in Colchester. A special ward was opened and there was no outside contact. Requirements were left at the door or window. Anything leaving the ward had to be burned immediately or stoved to disinfect it.

In the period 1936–39, a nurse described one smallpox patient's condition as 'ugly'. Another nurse, who did not care for any smallpox patients while training as a fever nurse at the City Hospital, Edinburgh (1938–41), 'specialled' a 2-year-old girl in her general training at the Victoria Hospital Glasgow (1941–44). The child, who was admitted in 1941 with a depressed fractured skull, was also a smallpox contact. She was later transferred to Ruchill Fever Hospital, Glasgow, and is believed to have survived. In 1947–49, a fever nurse probationer was sent out on ambulance duty to collect two smallpox patients who were, instead, found to be very ill children with chickenpox. Another nurse also mentioned a similar case of misdiagnosis. This common problem was generally averted in large hospitals as two doctors usually examined possible smallpox patients in the ambulance. However, a nurse at Fazakerley Hospital, Liverpool (1944–45), mentioned that 'one smallpox patient did get through; all nurses and patients were isolated in a ward'. In Bristol (1945–46), a probationer commented on how well the barrier nursing of smallpox patients was organised. 'All the nurses were volunteers and the medical officer, cook and cleaner lived in rooms above the ward'. Although staff were compulsorily isolated with patients, the duty attracted an extra payment and added leave which, together with the sense of camaraderie which developed, was some compensation for the incarceration and health risks involved.

The transmission of infectious diseases from one country to another has been an increasing problem since voyages of discovery were first made. As a result of travel within the British Empire in the nineteenth and much of the twentieth century, authorities in other countries provided care for British nationals who had contracted diseases abroad. Although outbreaks of small-pox were less frequent in Britain after 1901–02, the disease was still endemic in India and some other countries.

## Case history: a British family in India, 1928

Jean Crawford's account of a particularly serious outbreak of smallpox in Calcutta in 1928 is given here verbatim, to demonstrate the universal nature of care in this disease.

> I remember when I was six or seven years old in 1928 (I don't know the month), my mother, who was 32, had smallpox. My father T.J.Y. Roxburgh I.C.S. was Chief Presidency Magistrate Calcutta at the time. My mother and I had recently returned from home leave having left my brother at school in England. Daddy had returned from leave some months ahead of us. She and I had been vaccinated in England as always before returning to

India. I do not know how long we had been back, but it was considered recent enough for us not to be re-vaccinated when the municipal doctor came round to vaccinate the entire household. This was an annual event. We would all line up on the verandah, the sahib and memsahib and children first, and then the servants (all eight of them, the ayah probably first). I remember being told that there had been a particularly severe outbreak of smallpox in Calcutta that year. As soon as Mummy was diagnosed as having actually developed smallpox I was immediately re-vaccinated (as always on my thigh) and had a severe reaction.

My mother was taken off to the isolation hospital in north Calcutta in Upper Circular Road, some way away in a bazaar area. I was always told that she did not have the disease very badly but nevertheless it was as bad as a very severe attack of chickenpox. She told me that she was painted with some dark brown stuff which I think was to help prevent pock marks. Anyway she certainly wasn't scarred at all, except I think for one mark on a leg.

I do not know how long that she was in hospital but I remember being taken by Daddy on several occasions to see her from a distance. The hospital was in a big compound surrounded by a wall and once inside I remember driving past long low one storey buildings; these I imagine were separate wards. At the far side of the compound and behind another high wall was the VIP [very important person] isolation building, red brick and two storeys with the usual wide verandahs which were caged in with wire mesh. The building was quite near the wall with the compound road running alongside, where we parked the car (an open bull nosed Morris). I'm fairly sure I remember correctly that Mummy was the only patient in that building. There were no wards, all rooms being private. Each patient had their own day nurse and night nurse. We never went behind the wall and I remember standing in the roadway and waving to her when she came out of her room on to the verandah on the first floor. I know that I couldn't see the ground floor of the building from the road. I remember these visits were sometimes after dark, which was obviously after Daddy came back from Court, sunset being fairly early all the year round. Other recollections are the usual brilliant sunshine, which must have been weekend visits. I do not know how long it was after she went into hospital that I was taken to see her. She had no other visitors, except Padre Pearson, the Cathedral chaplain, who was actually allowed in to see her. That is all I can remember. My mother died at the end of 1982, aged 86.[104]

A number of issues arise from this account including the risk to the family of being in close contact with what were then termed 'native servants', who could transmit the disease to upper-class British families. Nowhere was the class system more rigidly upheld than in the British Empire. However, it is clear that this family took every precaution for themselves and for their staff to prevent smallpox, but the disease was so virulent in 1928 in Calcutta that it affected Jean's mother. The evidence shows that even recent vaccination did not protect her completely, although she had the mildest form, with only a small eruption of pocks, and she survived into old age. Isolation of the patient and visiting from a distance were typical of régimes in Britain then, apart from the one to one ratio of patient and nurse in the special treatment accorded to a private patient.

## Conclusion

This research has revealed a number of anomalies in the provision of care from the early eighteenth century, and a somewhat tardy approach by central government to a disease which was at its worst before relatively effective preventive measures were implemented. Hence, throughout the nineteenth century, many nurses working in general hospitals, asylums and workhouses were put at risk of contracting the disease inadvertently. Most late-nineteenth-century compulsory health legislation was intended to protect the health of the nation, but British resistance to compulsory vaccination of infants from 1898 meant that the population was still susceptible to contracting smallpox. Institutions were still needed and nurses and other health care workers were exposed to a disease which had been largely controlled in Germany. Probationers were recruited primarily for their labour and (as has been seen) training, which included theoretical aspects of the care of smallpox patients, was offered in fever hospitals, mainly to retain their services. Considering that the last major epidemic in Britain was in 1901–02, it took the nursing profession a long time to organise itself with regard to smallpox and other infectious diseases.

Smallpox hospitals were separate institutions or units. Probationers undergoing fever nurse training were seldom obliged to nurse patients with this disease, but most did so willingly if need arose. Nurses in small fever hospitals in remote areas were unlikely to meet the disease very often, if at all, whereas those in large cities and port areas were more likely to gain some clinical experience during their training. Without the nursing care so willingly given in smallpox hospitals, it is likely that the final outcome of many patients would have been more adversely affected. Nurses almost certainly saved some lives, and very likely prevented some disfigurement, blindness, and other complications, by their assiduous attention to the rash, to the eyes and the delirium. Should the disease break out again, as a result of bioterrorist activity, it would once again become primarily a nurses' disease as they would form the main workforce in the care of smallpox patients. The issue of bioterrorism is discussed further in Chapter 8. It is only by learning from the past and having an awareness of current research and world affairs, that nurses, and the necessary support staff, would have a greater chance of survival in epidemic situations. Only then would they be able to provide that essential service required by society, good nursing care.

## Notes and references*

1 McKeown and Lowe (1974), p. 9, Table 2. Mean annual mortality rates per million living (standardised to age and sex distribution of 1901 population) due to certain communicable diseases in decennia 1851–60 and 1891–1900.
2 Hardy (1993), p. 110.
3 D. A. Henderson (1999) 'Smallpox Virus Destruction. The Research Agenda Utilizing Variola Virus: A Public Health Perspective', *Biodefense News*, December, http://www.hopkins-biodefense.org/pages/news/research.html (18 April 2000).
4 The Jenner Museum, Berkeley, Gloucester. Professor Reginald Shooter, chairman of the Government's Dangerous Pathogens Advisory Group (1975–81), was instrumental in assembling this international collection.
5 M. R. Currie (2001) 'Smallpox Nursing in Britain, Part II: Nursing Care and Nurse Training', *International History of Nursing Journal*, 6(2): 59–65.
6 Zimmerman and Zimmerman (2003), p. 214.
7 Henderson, op. cit.
8 Porter (1997), p. 486.
9 D. A. Henderson, Inglesby, T. V., Bartlett, J. G., Ascher, M. S., Eitzen, E., et al. (1999) 'Smallpox as a Biological Weapon: Medical and Public Health Management', *Journal of the American Medical Association*, 281(22): 2128.
10 D. A. Henderson (1999) 'About the First National Symposium on Medical and Public Health Response to Bioterrorism', *Emerging Infectious Diseases*, 5(4): 491. The other countries represented were Austria, Finland, Israel and Italy.
11 J. P. Robinson (1999) 'News Chronology: August through October 1999', *The CBW Conventions Bulletin*, 46 (December): 32.
12 Hardy (1993), p. 112.
13 Riddell (n.d.[1914]), p. 182.
14 Richardson (1998), p. 2.
15 Zimmerman and Zimmerman (2003), p. 9.
16 Hardy (1993), p. 114.
17 L. Dopson (1948) 'The Passing of the Poor Laws', *Nursing Times*, 3 July: 480.
18 Wesley (1960[1747]), pp. 103–04.
19 Buchan (1824[1769]), pp. 162–71.
20 Currie (1982), p. 14.
21 Richardson (1998), p. 55.
22 Bedfordshire and Luton Archives and Records Service (BLARS) P35/12/8 Papers relating to the Pest House at Caddington.
23 BLARS P35/12/3 Articles of agreement, Pest House at Caddington.
24 BLARS P35/5/1 Churchwardens Account Book, Parish of Caddington.
25 I am grateful to Stephen R. Coleman, Historic Environment Information Officer, Heritage and Environment Section, Bedfordshire County Council, for supplying a list of pesthouses currently known in Bedfordshire, 8 January 2003. The present owner, Mr Ray Attewell, kindly showed the Chalgrave Pesthouse to me on 9 February 2004.
26 Richardson (1998), p. 132.
27 Lane (2000), p. 59.

*———

Full references appear in the Bibliography.

28 C. D. Linnell (ed.) (1999) *Historical Carlton through the Diary of Benjamin Rogers, Rector of Carlton, 1720–1771*, Carlton and Chellington Historical Society. This is a reprint edition published by the society to commemorate the fiftieth anniversary of the original publication in 1949, pp. 14, 26.

29 Ibid., pp. 71, 88.

30 Woodforde (1978), pp. 395–97.

31 Monument from demolished Church, St James, Hampstead Road, London, now in the Victoria and Albert Museum, London. The marble is signed by John Bacon the Younger. Seen by the author, 20 November 2003.

32 Ranger and Slack (1992), pp. 159–160.

33 BLARS QSR 1731/94(A) Notes and Extracts in the Quarter Session Rolls, 1714–1832, Vol. I.

34 Lane (2000), p. 168.

35 Underwood (1974), p. 22.

36 BLARS PUAM/10 Minutes of the Board of Guardians, Ampthill Union.

37 BLARS PUAM/10 Meeting of the Ampthill Board of Guardians, 5 January 1882.

38 F.B. Smith (1979), p. 389.

39 Woodward (1974), pp. 52–53, 177.

40 Whitteridge and Stokes (1961), p. 35.

41 Selby-Green (1990), p. 50.

42 M.R. Currie (2001) 'Smallpox Nursing in Britain, Part I: Diseases, Patients, their Nurses and Places of Care', *International History of Nursing Journal* 6(1): 48–55.

43 LMA HL/B/MXJ, Middlesex Districts Joint Smallpox Hospital Board: Clare Hall Hospital. It was finally transferred to Clare Hall, South Mimms, in Middlesex in 1896.

44 Taylor (1991), p. 14.

45 Frazer (1950), p. 290.

46 Abel-Smith (1964), pp. 127–28.

47 LGB (1916) *Forty-fourth Annual Report of the Local Government Board 1914–1915, Part III – (a) Public Health and local Administration*, London: HMSO Cd 8197. See Table 2.2, p.20.

48 *Burdett's Hospitals and Charities Year Book, 1922–1923*.

49 Frazer (1950), p. 290.

50 See Abbreviations and common terms on p.xvi.

51 Coleman and Salt (1992), pp. 27–28.

52 J. M. Eyler (1976) 'Mortality Statistics and Victorian Health Policy', *Bulletin of the History of Medicine*, 50(3): 335–55.

53 Hardy (1993), p. 112.

54 Ayers (1971), pp. 27–28.

55 Ibid, pp. 125, 181, 188–89. In 1904 the camp and ships were replaced by permanent buildings. A hulk was an abandoned battleship, used in the nineteenth century as a prison or to isolate those with infectious diseases.

56 *Nursing Record*, 12 April 1888: 17–18.

57 Ibid., 19 April 1888: 30–31.

58 LMA MAB 1623, *Annual Report 1929–30*, p. 105.

59 Burne (1996), p. 61. See Ayers (1971), p. 147, re male staff.

60 A. Hardy (1983) 'Smallpox in London: Factors in the Decline of the Disease in the Nineteenth Century', *Medical History*, 27: 111–38.

61 LGB (1882) *Tenth Annual Report of the Local Government Board 1880–81*. Supplement

containing Reports and Papers submitted by the Board's Medical Officer on the Use and Influence of Hospitals for Infectious Diseases. C3290, London: HMSO.

62 Searle (1965), p. 68.

63 RCNA C370 The Local Authority of the City of Perth. Infectious Hospital, Friarton, Perth. Rules for Nurses, Ward Maids, etc., n.d. [1919], and *Burdett's Hospitals and Charities, 1922–23*.

64 Monk (1978), pp. 15–16.

65 LMA H/NW1/SP4 Smallpox and Vaccination Hospital, Register of In-patients, 4 April 1879 to 12 April 1905. A cicatrix is a scar, in this case from vaccination. Four good marks were considered satisfactory then.

66 LMA MAB/2636 MAB *Annual Report 1922*, Infectious Diseases Section, p. 75.

67 Burne (1996), p. 73. The patient records which should include this nurse are closed for 100 years. See LMA H48/B/01/113 Case Register (1 Volume) January 1919 – July 1929, closed until 2030.

68 Gray (1999), p. 212. See also Berkeley, Jenner Museum (BEKJM) /1564 *The Edinburgh Outbreak of Smallpox 1942*. City of Edinburgh Public Health Department, which includes patients' histories and treatments.

69 *Daily Telegraph*, 28 March 1950.

70 Ibid., 11 April 1950.

71 *Nursing Record*, 19 April 1888: 30–31. At that time, water beds were used to prevent bed sores in very ill patients. They comprised a fixed outer covering of strong rubber almost filled with water.

72 Berkeley, Jenner Museum (BEKJM)0169 Case 4129a (Elizabeth Slade) from the bound volume of MAB hospital ship *Castalia*, the Nurses' Reports and Smallpox Cases Bed Cards (cases 4101a–4220a).

73 Ayers (1971), pp. 282–83.

74 Sworder (1893).

75 RCNA (Historic Pamphlet Collection 3B), 'Isla Stewart: her Life, and her Influence on the Nursing Profession'. First memorial oration by Miss Rachael Cox-Davies, London: The National Council of Trained Nurses of Great Britain and Ireland, 24 November 1911.

76 BEKJM/412/42 'The Story of the Smallpox Epidemic in Middlesbrough', *Northern Weekly Gazette*, Middlesbrough, 1898.

77 Watson (1945), p. 190.

78 McCleary (1935), p. 133. Six candidates received the certificate. By the end of 1900, the annual number of candidates had risen to 929. By then, 5,529 midwives had received the certificate.

79 'My Life, By An Old Nurse', *Nursing Times*, 16 October 1926: 922–25.

80 F. B. Smith (1979), p. 160.

81 Gray (1999), pp. 147–48, 431.

82 Annual Report, County MOH, Durham, 1902, xi–xii. Hardy (1993), pp. 144–47, discusses concerns about the persistence of the disease in the vagrant population in late-nineteenth-century London.

83 Annual Report, School Medical Officer, Borough of Luton, 1909.

84 Chief Constable's Report, Borough of Luton, 1909.

85 Currie (1982), p. 46.

86 Borough of Luton, Council Minutes and Reports, Council Meeting, 20 March 1928.

87  Currie (1982), p. 41. In an interview with Mrs Bracey in 1982, she remembered it as 'about 1929'.
88  Borough of Luton Council Minutes, Council Meeting, 31 July 1928.
89  Annual Report, MOH, Luton, 1932.
90  North East Lincolnshire Archives (NELA) Annual Report, MOH, County Borough of Grimsby, 1947, pp. 44–47.
91  Ibid.
92  NELA 'The Medical Officer of Health's report on the outbreak of smallpox, April 14th, 1947 to the Health Committee'. County Borough of Grimsby.
93  *Nursing Record and Hospital World*, 7 June 1902.
94  *BJN*, 21 August 1909: 158.
95  *BJN*, 23 May 1914: 462.
96  See for example 'Syllabus of Subjects for Examination for the Certificate of General Nursing'. GNC for England and Wales, 1923.
97  Pearce (1940).
98  Woolacott (1906), pp. iii, 88, 97.
99  Riddell (n.d.[1914]), pp. 182–83.
100  Watson (1939), pp. 159–68.
101  Ibid.
102  Hardy, 'Smallpox in London', op. cit., p. 131.
103  M. R. Currie (1997–8) 'Fever Nurses' Perceptions of their Fever Nurse Training, 1921–71'. *International History of Nursing Journal*, 3(2): 13–14, and Currie, 'Smallpox Nursing in Britain Part I', op. cit., 48–55.
104  BEKJM/560/3 Testimony of Jean Crawford, June 1992.

# 6    Fever Nurse Cavell in the 1890s

Edith Cavell ... an outstanding British patriot ... a very brave woman.
A. E. Clark-Kennedy (1965)[1]

## Introduction

Edith Louisa Cavell (1865–1915) is known by most people as the nurse who was shot dead by the Germans in Brussels in the First World War on 12 October 1915, for helping over 200 Belgian, French and British soldiers to escape, despite knowing that she had nursed German wounded.[2] What is less well known is that she was an artist of no mean ability, and that she was a fever nurse in London in the late nineteenth century (Figure 6.1).[3]

Her reasons for taking up this kind of work have been discussed from various perspectives, albeit very briefly. For example, in 1965, Archibald E. Clark-Kennedy, Physician to the London Hospital in Whitechapel (1927–58), where Edith undertook a general nurse training course (1896–98), presented his rationale from a medical viewpoint. He noted that nursing in a fever hospital was a much tougher proposition in the 1890s than it was in the 1960s. Diphtheria was still common, a high cause of mortality in children; although antitoxin had just been introduced, there was no prophylactic inoculation. Many cases of laryngeal diphtheria, the most serious form of the disease, required tracheotomy (an artificial opening into the trachea, carried out as an emergency to allow the patient to breathe). Scarlet fever was serious, often resulting in renal and mastoid complications. Measles was also dangerous, as many children developed broncho-pneumonia and without antibiotics had a very high mortality rate.[4] It is clear then, that at that time, such work was no sinecure.

It is important, therefore, to consider more closely why Edith, an educated, relatively independent, middle-class woman, should want, at nearly 30 years of age, to enter an environment where children were often gravely ill, suffering and frequently dying. Born to the Reverend Frederick and Louisa Sophia Cavell at Swardeston, five miles south of Norwich, she was the first of four children: Edith (4 December 1865), Florence (1867), Lilian (1870) and John, known as Jack (1873). The oldest child in a family often matures more

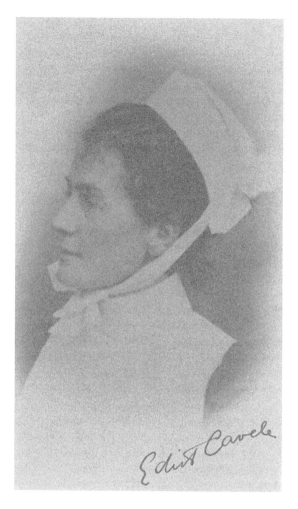

*Figure 6.1* Edith Cavell,
Night Sister, St Pancras
Infirmary, 1901–03.
Royal London Hospital
Archives

quickly than the others, frequently with a sense of responsibility to younger siblings. Moreover, as a vicar's daughter, Edith was conscious of her Christian duty to others. She grew up knowing everyone in the parish and regularly took hot meals from the family table to those less fortunate, particularly the aged, those 'in trouble, sorrow, need, sickness or any other adversity'.[5] Although she was to face adversity herself at times, the worst was, undoubtedly, the situation she met in Brussels in the First World War. Ironically, her name means 'happy in war'.[6] However, this period of her life was, as yet, quite distant.

Her growing independent spirit could be seen in the way she campaigned for a Sunday school in Swardeston. At 20 years of age, on her own initiative, she wrote to the Bishop of Norwich, John Thomas Pelham, suggesting that episcopal help was needed. He replied that, if the village could raise a certain amount of money, he would see what could be done about the remainder. Not easily thwarted, Edith helped raise the necessary funds by selling her artwork: pencil sketches, water-colour paintings and the Christmas cards she had made, with the help of her family. The new building was opened two years later in 1888.[7] During her childhood, and on visits back to Swardeston, from various posts she held as a governess in England, and in Belgium, where she spent five years (1890–95), she visited parishioners at home and saw the problems experienced by mothers trying to care for sick children, some perhaps, with infectious diseases. Her unexpected return from Brussels to nurse her father in June 1895 is often given as the reason for her wanting to take up nursing. Although this may have been the case, it is unlikely to have been the only reason.

## Social conscience

It was probably at about this time that she became more aware of the importance of public opinion in England and began to consider current beliefs and practices with regard to the poor and the sick. It is likely that she knew of Samuel Smiles' 1859 doctrine of self-help, which was designed to show what could be accomplished by determination and the will to succeed.[8] Although his work was extremely popular for some years and achieved international publicity, its influence had largely faded by the 1890s. It had done little for those in grinding poverty, unable to help themselves and may even have exacerbated the contemporary idea that the poor were deservedly so, a belief enshrined in the punitive Poor Law Amendment Act, 1834, parts of which were still in force in the 1890s.

Edith would also have known of the pioneering initiatives of female social reformers, such as Elizabeth Fry (1780–1845), the Quaker prison reformer, Louisa Twining (1820–1912), who campaigned for trained nurses for the workhouse sick in separate infirmaries, and Octavia Hill (1838–1912), who worked among the poor in London improving the homes of people in the slums. Elizabeth Garrett Anderson (1836–1917), one of the first female doctors, recognised the poor health problems of women and opened a dispensary for them in London in 1866, later renamed the Elizabeth Garrett Anderson Hospital. In 1870, Elizabeth was appointed a visiting physician to the East London Hospital. She also supported her sister, the equally redoubtable Millicent Fawcett, in the moderate suffragist movement.

Probably the most significant person from Edith's perspective was Florence Nightingale (1820–1910), nationally and internationally known for her work in the Crimean War (1854–56), and her subsequent efforts to improve the status and training of nurses.[9] The work carried out by 'the great and the good' would have provided some interesting points for her father's long sermons, discussion in the family and quiet reflection. Edith's father graduated in theology from King's College London and then studied at Heidelberg, before being ordained. While abroad, he may have read and discussed Frederick Engels' *The Condition of the Working Class in England, From*

*Personal Observation and Authentic Sources*, which was published in Germany in 1845 and the United States in 1887, but was not published in London until 1892, because of its inflammatory nature. During his curacy in London, at St Mark's Church, Islington, he would have been exposed to the plight of the sick and been aware of the street urchins who roamed the streets, many of whom were orphaned.

There were certainly opportunities for help to be given, especially in the East End of London. where the condition of the poor had long been strikingly obvious to those who frequented the warrens of streets with squalid dwellings. The 'Condition of England' novels, which were part of a literary genre begun by Thomas Carlyle in *Chartism* (1830) and *Past and Present* (1843), highlighted the problems and heralded Benjamin Disraeli's *Sibyl or The Two Nations* (1845), which described 'the Condition of the People' and contrasted the lives of the rich and poor in England, as did Charles Dickens' *Hard Times* (1854).

The Cavell family would almost certainly have been familiar with these books, which may have stirred the conscience of some people. Thomas Barnado (1845–1905), who qualified as a doctor at the London Hospital, not only helped local children by becoming the Superintendent of a 'ragged school' (a free school for poor children), but also set up homes for waifs and strays previously roaming the streets: boys in 1870, and girls in 1876. Those children were noticed because of their visibility, unlike those in their own homes where cruelty, including neglect, often went undetected. It was not until as late as 1884, however, that the National Society for the Prevention of Cruelty to Children opened a branch in London, a year after the first one established in Liverpool, based on the New York model.[10]

It was mostly the intellectuals, the educated middle and upper classes, who railed against these circumstances and largely shaped public opinion; in some cases, like Barnado, they resorted to deeds, rather than just words. University students, initially from Oxford, played a big part in social work among the poor in the East End of London, where help was most needed. Toynbee Hall, named after Arnold Toynbee (1852–83), was opened in Commercial Street, Whitechapel, with the Reverend Samuel A. Barnet (1844–1913), the Vicar of St Jude's, Whitechapel, as warden in 1884. This, the first university settlement, did much good work among the poor in the district. University men, who went into residence to take part in social work, helped to create a centre of popular education and recreation.

Different aspects of people's lives received attention, but the charitable impulse was mostly haphazard and uncoordinated, although it paved the way for increased state intervention. Nevertheless, it was the good works by individuals and groups, often motivated by religious beliefs and, for some, a sense of *noblesse oblige*,[11] which played a large part in changing social conscience in England by the time Edith was ready to become a nurse in the mid-1890s. There was considerable precedent, therefore, for work with the poor and the sick in London's most deprived districts. This factor was probably paramount in her mind and greatly influenced her decision to apply for a general nurse training course at the London Hospital in Whitechapel, which had opened a 'training establishment' in 1873,[12] and the first preliminary training school in England in 1895. There she would receive a six-week course, away from the wards, learning practical nursing skills and sickroom cookery, and attending lectures on elementary anatomy, physiology and hygiene. During the seventh week she would be examined in these subjects.[13]

Before this, however, Edith needed to try out this new profession, to test her vocation and see if she could fit in with living and working in a large organisation. What better than to begin in a fever hospital where the patients were predominantly needy children? It would probably have seemed a relatively easy step from managing and educating children to caring for them in sickness. Edith had already broken away from home to take governess posts in England and in Belgium; perhaps her vocation was really in nursing, by then a more acceptable and respected occupation.

## Pandemic of influenza in Europe and North America

While Edith was working in Brussels in the early 1890s, she would probably have been aware of the pandemic of influenza 1889–92, which swept across Europe, Britain and North America. She almost certainly knew about the epidemic of Asiatic cholera in Europe, which decimated Hamburg in Germany and caused alarm in London, where an epidemic of scarlet fever was already at its height. In 1893, a recrudescence of scarlet fever and an outbreak of smallpox, plus the threat of cholera and influenza led to the need for more accommodation for the infectious sick in London. A hastily constructed 'makeshift hospital', the 'Fountain', opened in Tooting, South London in 1893.[14] The six MAB fever hospitals had admitted 14,500 patients in 1893, but 6,000 were refused admission due to a shortage of beds. When the public became aware of these facts and of the continued high incidence of scarlet fever, a number of questions were asked in Parliament between June and September 1895, which resulted in more land being made available to the MAB. Within a few months, three more fever hospitals, the 'Park' at Lewisham, the 'Grove' at Tooting (opposite the Fountain), and the 'Brook' at Woolwich, all in the growing districts of south London, were under construction to add to those already managed by the MAB.[15]

## New fever hospitals in London and recruitment problems

The proposed establishment of infectious disease (fever) hospitals in heavily populated districts, particularly those for smallpox, caused panic and resulted in public inquiries as residents were fearful of the spread of infection. Although the MAB eventually solved this problem by building on the periphery of the metropolis and by using ships in the Thames' estuary for smallpox, it had another concern. The retention of nursing staff was essential if all its hospitals were to be run efficiently and patient care carried out properly.

In 1892, at the request of the MAB, Dr J. H. Bridges of the Local Government Board,[16] carried out a detailed study of the nursing situation in their hospitals. He found a general lack of trained staff. For example, only one of the nineteen charge nurses was fully trained and a number were under 20 years of age. Although untrained, some had had previous experience in workhouse sick wards, but relatively few had undergone a regular course of instruction at a hospital or at one of the eighteen Poor Law infirmaries in England which could be termed 'schools for nurses'. His investigation resulted in important reforms. He recommended that nursing staff should be treated as a class separate from, and superior to, other female subordinate staff, and that they be boarded and lodged apart from them. Nurses should have a separate bedroom and access to a comfortable, roomy sitting room. Pay was increased at once, and there were to be two grades of assistant nurse, Class I and Class II, the lower grade for inexperienced nurses.[17]

## Fever nursing at the Fountain Hospital

Edith was to benefit from these improvements as a Class II fever nurse at the Fountain Hospital. In order to give an insight into the well-ordered but confined world into which Edith would be committing herself, where she, not her pupils, was expected to be obedient, a detailed explanation of her new surroundings is necessary. The Fountain was only two years old when Edith began her nursing career there in 1895. It had been erected by the MAB as a temporary fever hospital on a ten-acre site purchased for £4,395 in 1893 in Tooting, South London (Figure 6.2). The Fountain was the first hospital to be established since Dr Bridges' report of 1892. The MAB clearly took his suggestions seriously, despite the so-called 'temporary' nature of the new hospital. It was designed in a pavilion-plan arrangement with sixteen rectangular, single-storey, twenty-four-bedded ward huts, identical in design, approached from a covered way by a short corridor, on one side of which was the ward scullery and the attendant's bedroom. On the other side was the linen room, staff lavatory and patients' bathroom. Adequate ventilation and sunlight was ensured by the large sash windows, which had hopper-hung fanlights. There was also an extractor fan in the ceiling. The sanitary arrangements were situated in the centre of the ward via a lobby. There were also two isolation blocks, located at the north-eastern edge of the site, and a workshop, boiler house and laundry.

The staff quarters, situated on the south-eastern border of the site, comprised four separate blocks for the different classes of nurses, each with a central corridor with single bedrooms or cubicles, according to the class of nurse, on either side. Bathrooms and lavatories were also provided. A fifth block contained the nurses' recreation room. There were also three huts to

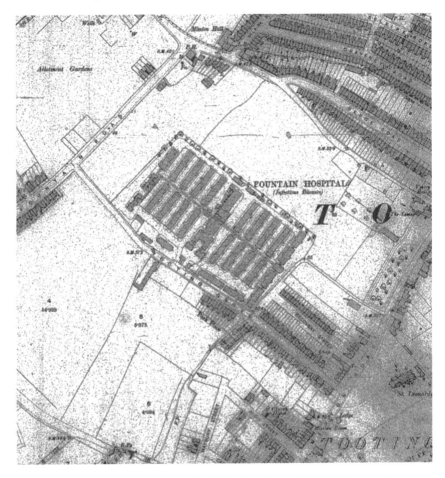

*Figure 6.2* Site plan, Fountain Hospital, Tooting Grove, 1897. Ordnance Survey,
Map Library, British Library

accommodate the seventy-six female domestics and a further hut near the
hospital entrance housed the male servants. The administrative offices,
which faced the entrance gates, were at the centre of the site. There was also
a porter's lodge facing Tooting Grove with a gate office, waiting room and a
lavatory with 'discharging rooms' and bathrooms at the rear. The lodge had
gates on either side, one set forming an 'infected entrance' leading to the
receiving wards and the other set forming a 'non-infected' entrance leading
to the administration buildings and stores. The Matron and the Medical
Superintendent were situated in detached buildings on either side of a
central storage yard. A single-storey, brick-built mortuary contained a
viewing room, a post-mortem room and a 'body holders' room in between.
The mortuary yard was screened off by high brick walls and separate
entrance gates were provided in the boundary wall. The new hospital,

designed by Thomas W. Aldwinckle, the MAB architect, was erected and completely furnished in nine weeks at a cost of £120,000, and opened in October 1893, supplying 400 additional fever beds.[18]

Dr Caiger, Medical Superintendent of the Fountain, thought it hardly appropriate to call it a 'temporary building'. The walls may have been constructed of wood and iron, not bricks and mortar, but 'the foundations, drainage, machinery, steam, gas and water supplies and internal fittings are as sound in construction and as permanent' as in any similar institution, built of brick. The wards are well heated, bright and cheerful and benefit greatly from a width of 26 feet (7.92 metres), instead of 24 feet (7.32 m). Each bed has a space of 2,000 cubic ft (56.6 cu m).[19] The speed with which the Fountain was made ready for patients illustrates the efficiency of the MAB, which could respond so quickly to the urgent need for extra accommodation.

In its completeness, it was a world set apart from the community, similar to an asylum, what Ervine Goffman termed 'a total institution' where people were 'both incapable of looking after themselves and a threat to the community, albeit an unintentional one'.[20] It is very likely that Edith had tremendous misgivings about her new role as a fever nurse. Her lowly place in the hierarchy was almost certainly reinforced by her uniform as the most junior nurse and the allocation of a cubicle, not a bedroom, as befitted her new subordinate status. The lifestyle she had left was vastly different from hospital life, where she would be expected to carry out tasks quickly, obediently and without question. Nor had she probably realised that punctuality by the clock, as practised in elementary schools and factories, would be considered so important in nursing.[21]

Her application form to become an Assistant Nurse, Class II, at the Fountain, is dated 6 December 1895 (Figure 6.3).[22] As there was an immediate vacancy, she began only six days later on 12 December 1895.[23] It is clear, from what is now known about her, that Edith was not destined to fit into the role of junior nurse, following her responsible career as a governess. Her future was, as yet, not easy to envisage. Her brother, Jack, said later that, even as a young girl she seemed 'dominated and driven on by some inner sense of purpose'. She also told Margaret François, one of the four children she taught in Brussels, that her greatest ambition was 'to be buried in Westminster Abbey'. In a letter to her cousin Eddy in England, she wrote that her work as a governess was only temporary; some day she would do something *useful*. She did not know what it would be, but it would be something for people as most of them are 'so hopeless, so hurt, and so unhappy'.[24]

Apparently, a mere few months at the Fountain were enough to convince Edith that nursing was what she wanted to do with her life. Not only did it offer her a career where she could progress, if she wanted, but also it provided residential accommodation, an important benefit in London in the 1890s, as it was not socially acceptable for middle-class single women to live outside the family home. As the evidence relating to Edith Cavell's career at the Fountain is distinctly limited, it is necessary to enhance her profile by

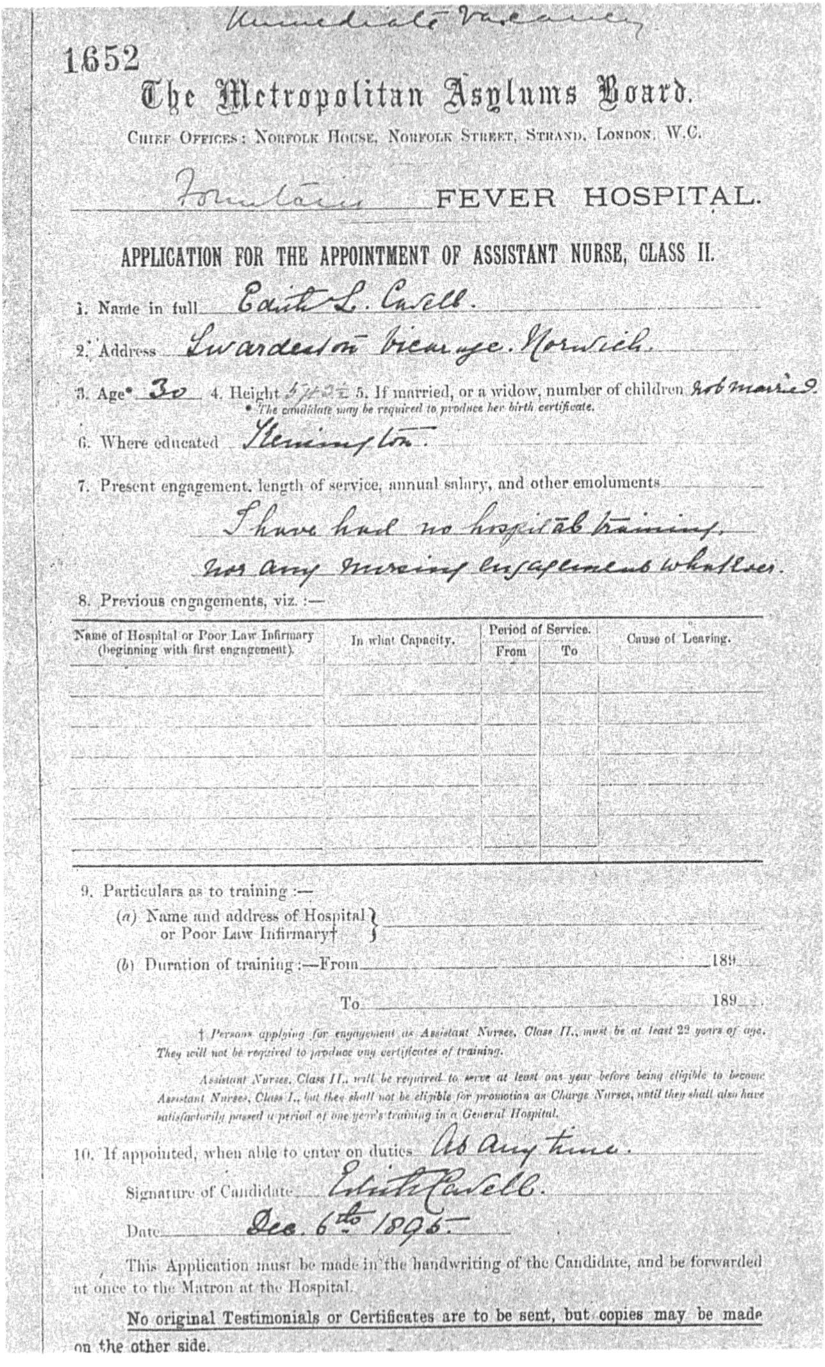
Immediate vacancy

1652

**The Metropolitan Asylums Board.**

CHIEF OFFICES: NORFOLK HOUSE, NORFOLK STREET, STRAND, LONDON, W.C.

Fountain FEVER HOSPITAL.

APPLICATION FOR THE APPOINTMENT OF ASSISTANT NURSE, CLASS II.

1. Name in full Edith L. Cavell.
2. Address Swardeston Vicarage. Norwich.
3. Age* 30 4. Height [illegible] 5. If married, or a widow, number of children not married.

* The candidate may be required to produce her birth certificate.

6. Where educated Kensington.
7. Present engagement, length of service, annual salary, and other emoluments

I have had no hospital training, nor any nursing engagement whatever.

8. Previous engagements, viz. :—

| Name of Hospital or Poor Law Infirmary (beginning with first engagement). | In what Capacity. | Period of Service. | | Cause of Leaving. |
|---|---|---|---|---|
| | | From | To | |
| | | | | |

9. Particulars as to training :—

(a) Name and address of Hospital or Poor Law Infirmary†

(b) Duration of training :—From 189

To 189

† Persons applying for engagement as Assistant Nurses, Class II., must be at least 22 years of age. They will not be required to produce any certificates of training.

Assistant Nurses, Class II., will be required to serve at least one year before being eligible to become Assistant Nurses, Class I., but they shall not be eligible for promotion as Charge Nurses, until they shall also have satisfactorily passed a period of one year's training in a General Hospital.

10. If appointed, when able to enter on duties At any time.

Signature of Candidate Edith Cavell.

Date Dec. 6th 1895.

This Application must be made in the handwriting of the Candidate, and be forwarded at once to the Matron at the Hospital.

**No original Testimonials or Certificates are to be sent, but copies may be made on the other side.**

*Figure 6.3* Edith Cavell's application form to be a fever nurse at the Fountain Hospital, 1895. London Metropolitan Archives using primary sources, purportedly concerning the London Hospital in Whitechapel, as some records held in their archives were written when she was still a fever nurse. It is unlikely that she would have changed much between April 1896, when she applied, and the time she began general nurse training at the London Hospital on 3 September 1896.

Some paying probationers were accepted there, but it was initially only for a period of three months and a fee of 13 guineas (£13.65) was payable. Edith was clearly a lady, but had already been earning her own living and probably needed the regular payment made to probationers of £12 in the first year and £20 in the second year.[25] This was significantly less than she was receiving at the Fountain where, like other MAB fever hospitals, it was found necessary to pay a relatively high salary to attract women to work as nurses in hazardous circumstances, where they could contract life-threatening infectious diseases. The longer period of training that regular probationers undertook would be a further test of her resolve to make nursing her vocation.

The application form for the London Hospital was more searching than that of the Fountain, and more important data about her are revealed in the professional and character references, which provide an insight into her work at the Fountain and her personal life. Edith completed the form on 17 April 1896 and then had to be interviewed. Much of the preliminary information is the same on the two application forms, although her height is now given as being 5ft 3inches (1.6m) and weight 8 stone (50.8 kg), therefore, of average build. She averred that she was strong, had always had good health and was possessed of perfect sight and hearing. She had been vaccinated against smallpox fourteen years previously and was apparently, according to a note in different writing, revaccinated on 4 May 1896. The only infectious diseases she had contracted were measles and whooping cough, but it is not known when or where she had these illnesses. Edith had not had rheumatism, rheumatic fever or varicose veins, conditions which could preclude, or severely hamper, a career in nursing. The form required her to state if she was a single woman or widowed, the assumption being that a married woman was unacceptable as a probationer, due to the obligatory residential criterion. She was happy to accept the vacancy on 18 July,[26] but did not, in fact, commence at the London until 3 September 1896.

Her Matron at the Fountain, Miss Dickenson, in a professional reference to Miss Eva Lückes, Matron of the London Hospital, was relatively brief and guarded in her remarks about her and her suitability for this employment. She wrote on 25 April 1896 that she had known 'Edith Cavill' [*sic*] since December 1895, but gave no details of her previous history, especially for the last three or four years as requested, presumably because she did not know. Her health was good, she was 'Orderly Methodical & of kindly & gentle disposition' with an equable temper and very pleasant manner. She was 'well educated, intelligent & capable', of good moral character and her work was carried out 'satisfactorily'. As Miss Dickenson had seen her daily in the wards she felt that Edith Cavill [*sic*] was 'a very suitable candidate for training as a hospital nurse'.[27] Edith may have appeared an ideal candidate for the London, but the guarded remark regarding practical work which, because of the emphasis on hygienic conditions, involved a lot of cleaning, did not augur well for her general training. She may have been destined for a post with greater responsibility, but she first had to endure the life of a lowly probationer.

A near neighbour in Norfolk, Mrs Annette Roberts of Brinton Hall, East Dereham, provided a personal reference on 27 April 1896. It gives a further insight into Edith's character. She stated that she had known her for fifteen years, declared her health was good and that she was energetic and ready to adapt herself to circumstances. Her intelligence was good and she was decidedly capable; her moral character was of high tone and she had a good deal of self-reliance. She thought that Edith was ready and, as far as she could judge, willing to follow guidance. In fact, Mrs Roberts had always had a high opinion of her and was glad of the opportunity of doing her a service and recommending her for the post as a regular probationer.[28] However, self-reliance was not necessarily an attribute expected at this stage of her career; it could alienate her from more senior nurses.

The terms and conditions of service in which nurses were employed in MAB fever hospitals, laid down after Dr Bridges' report in 1892, remained virtually the same for some years, apart from lowering the age of applicants. They would, therefore, have applied to Edith at the Fountain Hospital, where she nursed as an Assistant Nurse, Class II, for seven months from December 1895 until July 1896.

*Assistant Nurses, Class II.* – Applicants must be at least 22 years of age; must produce satisfactory evidence as to character, fair education, health, and physique, but are not required to hold certificates of previous training.

After a personal interview with the medical superintendent or matron, nurses are appointed by the Committees of Management of the hospitals. RECREATION, 12 hours weekly ; 1 day monthly ; evening passes may be granted when convenient, and are not counted in the 12 hours' leave, from 8.30 to 10 PM ; charge nurses, 4 weeks' holiday ; assistant nurses, 3 weeks' holiday in a year. All nurses are required to take a bath and change their uniform and stockings before going out of the hospitals. Nurses are subject to the authority of the matron and medical superintendents. Assistant nurses must obey the charge nurses under whom they work and from whom they receive instruction in practical ward work, and the nursing of infectious diseases. LECTURES are given in some of the hospitals by the medical superintendents or matrons. Testimonials are granted to all nurses after satisfactorily completing engagements of six months or longer. Assistant nurses, Class II, are eligible for promotion to Class I, but before they can be made charge nurses, they must obtain the 1 year's hospital experience required of assistant nurses, Class I, in addition to 2 years' service of the Board in fever nursing. Promotion and increase of salary in all cases depend upon the report of the medical superintendent and matrons concerned. SALARIES, charge nurses, £36, rising £1 annually to £40 per annum ; assistant nurses, Class I, £24, rising £1 annually to £28 per annum ; Class II, £20, rising £1 annually to £24 per annum.[29]

The Fountain was not a fever training hospital in the 1890s, although the clinical experience she gained there, with perhaps some lectures, would have given her a good grounding in basic nursing care and the bonus of a testimonial, as she was employed by the MAB for at least six months. Before hospitals issued their own nurse training certificates, they carried great weight and helped to ensure further employment, as long as they were positive.

Work in fever hospitals was not without risks. In 1895, Grace Rawlins, 'a young and promising assistant nurse' at the Fountain, died from pneumonia. In fact, 74 members of staff were warded that year with various complaints: '3 charge nurses, 5 assistant nurses and 1 ward maid contracted Scarlet Fever and 3 charge nurses, 3 assistant nurses and 4 ward maids contracted Diphtheria', all of whom recovered.[30] Edith would, perhaps, therefore have been pleased to acquire an insight into the new science of bacteriology, including the diagnostic development of the Klebs Löffler bacillus and the newly discovered antitoxic serum treatment for patients admitted with diphtheria in London.[31] MAB fever hospitals pioneered this treatment at the Eastern and the Fountain from 1894.[32] In 1895, antitoxin was given only to severe cases, but the loss of only one out of fourteen cases of diphtheria 'is an extremely satisfactory result'. The use of the new serum, and its success, was of overwhelming interest to the public and to the medical profession.[33]

The MAB had had a land ambulance service since 1881; Edith would, therefore, have witnessed horse-drawn ambulances arriving at the Fountain with patients being admitted with common conditions such as scarlet fever, diphtheria, enteric (typhoid) fever and, perhaps, some with typhus.[34] No account of the nursing care has been found during Edith's time at this hospital, but a description has survived of a similar MAB fever hospital a few years earlier. Dan Astley Gresswell, a young Oxford graduate, worked at the South-Western during the scarlet fever epidemic in 1887–88. Anne Hardy, the medical historian, thought it gave 'a rare insight into the realities of a MAB hospital ward'. She could detect the gentle approach of Charles West, the founder of Great Ormond Street Hospital, with the emphasis on cleanliness, rest and nourishment in Dan's account. On admission, patients with scarlet fever, who came from very poor backgrounds, were dressed in two bed-gowns, cotton underneath and flannel on top, before being put to bed in an airy ward with alternate upper small windows open all the time. Whatever the weather outside, an effort was made to maintain the temperature at 60° Fahrenheit (21°C).[35]

The iron beds had a feather mattress with a blanket and sheet under the patient, and a sheet, three blankets (more if requested), and a counterpane on top. Following admission, patients were all confined to bed for twenty-two days and, unless transferred to a convalescent hospital, remained in hospital for a minimum of eight weeks. Any amount of milk was permitted, plus eggs and ten ounces of beef tea daily, for the first twenty-two days. Although baths were not usually given in the first three weeks, once patients 'had been up for three or four days warm baths were given every evening before bed'. Relatively few medicines were used. Local applications of mustard (presumably in a poultice) were occasionally applied over enlarged cervical glands, but the main attention seems to have been directed to keeping the bowels open; Colocynth, castor oil and tinctures of Catechu and Kino were mentioned. A placebo, 'two or three drops of Spiritus Chloroformi to three ounces of water' was sometimes administered during the day, and in October and November, when complications were known to increase. A few patients received oxygen inhalations and oxygenated water, and when conditions such as heart weakness, softness of pulse and 'lividity of surface' were detected, port and brandy were administered.[36]

It is unlikely that much had changed in the care of scarlet fever patients when Edith began nursing at the Fountain seven years later, by which time the resistance and prejudice against hospitalisation of children, in some parts of London, had largely subsided.[37] Gwendoline M. Ayers' seminal work about the MAB provides quantitative data about the admission, and hospital case fatality percentage rates, of infectious diseases in their hospitals. Although it is not possible to distinguish the Fountain, from the other six fever hospitals in existence, while Edith was there (December 1895 to July 1896), it is likely that Edith would have nursed some of the very ill and dying patients, whose data are included in Table 6.1.

Scarlet fever, diphtheria and enteric (typhoid fever) were the most common notifiable infectious diseases treated in the MAB fever hospitals in the quinquennial period cited. The increased number of cases from 1896 was mainly due to the opening of the Brook in August that year and the Park in November 1897, which provided much needed extra accommodation for fever patients, but increased the demand for nursing staff. One factor is particularly significant, the fall in the hospital case fatality rate, particularly marked in diphtheria, once the new antitoxic serum had begun to take effect. It also shows the small number of admissions of patients with enteric in comparison to scarlet fever and diphtheria, although the hospital case fatality rate was much higher than in scarlet fever. Hardy has credited the decline in typhoid death rates in England and Wales, and London towards the end of the nineteenth century, to an upsurge of sanitary awareness with individual observation of the basic laws of hygiene, satisfactory water supplies and sewage disposal.[38] These factors were taken into account when other fever hospitals were established, and help to justify the emphasis placed on hygienic practices in nursing.

It is evident from the annual report of the Fountain Hospital in 1896 that it was a very busy institution. Many of the patients were dangerously ill on

Table 6.1 Patients admitted to **MAB** fever hospitals with certain infectious diseases, 1894–98

| Year | Admissions | | | Deaths | | | Hospital case fatality rate (%) | | |
|---|---|---|---|---|---|---|---|---|---|
| | Scarlet fever | Diphtheria | Enteric (typhoid fever) | Scarlet fever | Diphtheria | Enteric (typhoid fever) | Scarlet fever | Diphtheria | Enteric (typhoid fever) |
| 1894 | 11,598 | 3,666 | 534 | 717 | 1,035 | 96 | 5.92 | 29.29 | 18.13 |
| 1895 | 11,271 | 3,635 | 661 | 591 | 820 | 119 | 5.45 | 22.85 | 18.17 |
| 1896 | 15,982 | 4,508 | 600 | 666 | 948 | 96 | 4.29 | 21.2 | 15.84 |
| 1897 | 15,113 | 5,673 | 664 | 619 | 987 | 124 | 4.07 | 17.69 | 18.64 |
| 1898 | 12,125 | 6,566 | 869 | 514 | 991 | 143 | 4.12 | 15.37 | 17.73 |

Source: G. M. Ayers (1971) *England's First State Hospitals and the Metropolitan Asylums Board, 1867–1930*, London: Wellcome Institute of the History of Medicine, pp. 286–87.

admission, which meant Edith gained considerable experience in this specialism. The report includes data for the whole year, 1896, including statistics for diphtheria extracted for this study:

| | |
|---|---:|
| Patients remaining in hospital 31 December 1895 | 408 |
| Admissions in 1896 | 3,232 |
| Total number of patients under treatment in 1896 | 3,640 |
| (an increase of 1,178 admissions in 1895) | |
|     Discharged recovered | 1,335 |
|     Transferred to MAB Convalescent Hospital | 1,655 |
|     Died | 278 |
|     Remaining in hospital 31 December 1896 | 372 |
| Gross mortality on Registrar General's formula | 8.55% |
| (previous year 8.91%) | |
| Patients treated with diphtheria | 979 |
|     Discharged and recovered | 547 |
|     Transferred to another MAB hospital | 156 |
|     Died | 172 |
|     Remaining in hospital at end of year | 104 |

The Fountain managed to admit so many patients, the majority of whom were drawn from Wandsworth and Clapham, Lambeth, Camberwell and St James, because it had an MAB Convalescent Hospital available, to which some patients could be transferred. Of the 3,232 admissions in 1896, 107 (3.31 per cent) were not suffering from the disease for which they had been certified. The errors were 1.4 per cent in scarlet fever and 8.6 per cent in diphtheria cases. As was seen earlier, this could well have put hospital staff at risk, and definitely patients, as following admission, 66 cases contracted scarlet fever, of whom 13 died. It is also clear that some patients were sent in too late, as 40 of the 172 deaths due to diphtheria took place within 48 hours of admission. Nevertheless, there was room for optimism. There had been a considerable reduction in mortality in cases of diphtheria in 1895–96, in which antitoxin had been used. Before the use of antitoxin in MAB hospitals the mortality rate had been 30.3 per cent; in 1895 it was reduced to 19.47 per cent and in 1896 to 19.72 per cent. Had 'the patients arrived at the hospital earlier in their disease, and not, as was often the case, in a moribund condition, the results would have been even more striking than they are'. Nevertheless, there was now a 'feeling of hopefulness in doctor and nurse alike' in the treatment of laryngeal diphtheria.[39]

## Fever experience in general training and her subsequent career

The experience Edith gained at the Fountain served her in good stead in her subsequent general training at the London Hospital, which began in

September 1896. It included care of some patients with infectious diseases, and those in the typhoid epidemic at Maidstone, where she (and others) had been sent to help in 1897. Although not fully trained, Edith, apparently, acquitted herself well. Miss Lückes wrote that 'she did good work during the typhoid epidemic at Maidstone'; she thought Edith 'had a self-sufficient manner, which was very apt to prejudice people against her' and was 'best fitted for the Private Nursing Staff' in her third year of service.[40] This decision had a twofold benefit, first for the London. In 1886, Miss Lückes had started a private nursing institution attached to the hospital; the fees charged were two guineas (£2.10) weekly, rising to three guineas (£3.15) after an eight-week attendance.[41]

Miss Lückes tended to select the more self-sufficient probationers for private cases. Such work augmented the coffers of this voluntary hospital, but profit was not the only motive. The Maidstone typhoid epidemic was an emergency, and nurses rallied round to help each other. The second benefit was to Edith herself, as private nursing almost certainly improved her knowledge, skills and attitudes to patients in different settings, although she usually returned to the hospital between cases. It also enabled her to act on her own initiative to a greater extent than was possible in hospital. From October 1898 until December 1899, when she was appointed staff nurse in Mellish Ward at the London Hospital, she worked under the auspices of the London Hospital Private Nursing Institution. Her private patients included a 14-year-old boy in West Norwood, London, suffering from typhoid, who recovered after twelve weeks, a gentlemen with an inoperable carcinoma in Sussex, a lady with pleurisy and pneumonia in Lower Tottenham, London, and another case of inoperable cancer at Woburn, Bedfordshire.[42] Her previous experience of nursing patients with infectious diseases, particularly at the Fountain, would also have been invaluable during her time in positions of responsibility at Poor Law institutions in London as Night Superintendent at the St Pancras Infirmary (1901–03) and Assistant Matron at Shoreditch Infirmary, Hoxton (1903–06),[43] where patients with infectious diseases were still to be found. Apparently, she was not only a very efficient officer, but was 'much loved by the poor of Hoxton, amongst whom, in her off duty time, she did much good work'.[44]

In 1902, the Departmental Committee on Nursing the Sick Poor in Workhouses automatically approved infirmaries of a hundred beds and over as training schools.[45] As the St Pancras and Shoreditch infirmaries were large institutions, Edith would have gained experience in the training of probationers. According to Mary Caroline Day, one of sixty probationers at St Pancras, when Edith was one of two night sisters, she 'was so conscientious... to the nurses she was a true friend', but there was, 'just a touch of aloofness which perhaps in the interests of discipline is advisable'.[46] It may have been by chance, or due to her social conscience, that she elected to work in the infirmaries of these two particular London workhouses. They were mentioned by Engels in 1845 in *The Condition of the Working Class in England*, because of the appallingly bad, but not unusual, working practices which took place in the mid-1840s. They were unlikely, however, to have come to Edith's attention until after 1892, when the book was first published in England. Many of the facts made disturbing reading. For instance, in St Pancras Workhouse an epileptic died of suffocation during a fit; no one came to his aid. He could have been bound tight to his bed to save the nurses the trouble of sitting up at night – a practice known to have caused a death in Bacton, Suffolk, in January 1844. At St Pancras Workhouse, four, six or even eight children slept in one bed, and at Shoreditch Workhouse, a man and a fever patient, who was violently ill, shared a bed which teemed with vermin.[47] It is unlikely that similar conditions still prevailed in London workhouse infirmaries in the first part of the twentieth century, mainly due to the movement for workhouse and Poor Law reform in the 1850s and 1860s in which Florence Nightingale, Louisa Twining and others were active.[48]

Edith's decision to consolidate her fever and general nursing experience by working as a trained nurse within the Poor Law, not in a voluntary hospital, showed her humanity; she was ready to care for, and manage the care of, anyone who needed her. The prestigious voluntary hospitals, staffed by well-known consultants, reliant on charitable donations and patronised by royalty, would not take cases of venereal disease, and at that time, the MAB fever hospitals often refused to admit cases of measles and whooping cough. Poor Law infirmaries were obliged to receive patients who were not welcome elsewhere, including those with pulmonary tuberculosis.[49] It is clear that Edith did not show prejudice to any patients or their diseases. For example, in 1904, she applied for the vacant post of Matron at the Consumption Hospital, Ventnor, Isle of Wight.[50] Increasingly, she was able to pass on her knowledge, skills and management experience to other nurses in the years before her career as Matron of the first training school for nurses, near Brussels in Belgium, was brought to an abrupt end in 1915, at the age of 49 years.

## Conclusion

It is now clear that her decision to work with the sick and needy at the Fountain, the London and in Poor Law infirmaries was largely dictated by her social conscience, for, as mentioned previously, she found most people, 'so hopeless, so hurt, and so unhappy'. Her general nursing career, her arrest and execution in 1915 have been well documented by a number of authors, virtually to the exclusion of the time she spent in fever nursing, yet the period December 1895 to July 1896 was a catalyst for change in her life, which set her on the path towards becoming a nurse leader. Edith Cavell, as has been seen, was not a typical fever nurse.

After the end of the First World War on 11 November 1918, arrangements were made for her body to be exhumed and brought back to England. Although Edith had hoped to be interred in Westminster Abbey, her sisters,

Florence and Lilian, felt that she should be buried in Norfolk. However, the first part of the burial service was held at the Abbey on 15 May 1919, before her coffin was transported by train from Liverpool Street Station to Norwich. She was laid to rest in Life's Green just outside the south transept of Norwich Cathedral, not far from her childhood home at Swardeston.[51]

It is unlikely she will be forgotten, particularly by nurses, as her name and deeds live on in many countries in commemorative plaques, roads, squares, buildings and other memorials. For instance, an annual service is held at the Glacier of the Angel at the foot of Mount Edith Cavell in the Jasper National Park, Alberta, Canada.[52] In London, the seat of her nursing knowledge and experience in fever and general nursing, more restraint is evident. A life-like statue, situated in St Martin's Place, overlooking Trafalgar Square, was unveiled by Queen Alexandra on 17 March 1920. In 1924, Edith Cavell's own words were added to the pedestal, 'Patriotism is not enough; I must have no hatred or bitterness for anyone.' Her fitting words are just as relevant in the twenty-first century where nurses continue to work in perilous conditions, seldom deterred by danger, famine, infectious disease or war.

## Notes and references*

1 Clark-Kennedy (1965), p. 233.
2 In fact she was sentenced for conducting soldiers to the enemy (Britain), which she had not done; she had merely arranged their passage to the Dutch border. What they did when they crossed the frontier was not Edith's responsibility. The sentence was, therefore, unjust. See Ryder (1975), p. 238.
3 Daunton (1990). This short book, illustrated with some of Edith Cavell's water-colours, commemorates the 75th anniversary of her death and the 250th anniversary of the London Hospital, which received the title 'Royal' in 1990.
4 Clark-Kennedy (1965), p. 28. Cases of measles and whooping cough were not officially admitted to MAB fever hospitals until 1911.
5 Ibid., p. 19.
6 Ibid., p. 3.
7 Ryder (1975), pp. 20–21.
8 Smiles (1860[1859]).
9 Baly (1995), p. 146. Many girls were named after Florence Nightingale, including, probably, Edith's own sister. Coincidentally, like Edith, Florence Nightingale did not begin her nursing career until she was 30 years old.
10 Behlmer (1982), pp. 52–3, 63, 72.
11 The supposed obligation of nobility to be honourable and generous.
12 Parker and Collins (1998), p. 20.
13 McGann (1992), pp. 19–20.
14 Ayers (1971), p. 97. The Fountain Fever Hospital, often mistakenly referred to as 'The Fountains', existed from 1893 to 1912 and then became the Fountain Mental

---
*Full references appear in the Bibliography.

Hospital from 1912 to 1948: Hospital Records Database: http://www.hospital-records.pro.gov.uk (accessed 12 June 2003). In 1911, the MAB removed the Fountain from its isolation hospitals' service and reallocated it as a mental hospital for the treatment of the lowest grade of severely subnormal children. With additions and alterations, this 'temporary' hospital survived until the early 1960s, when it was demolished to make way for the new St George's Hospital at Tooting (data from English Heritage, 10 October 2003). Ayers (1971) is mistaken about some information given about the Fountain. Although accurately mentioned as a fever hospital on p. 97, it is inaccurately cited on p. 276, where it is given as a mental hospital, opened in October 1893. Confusion about the Grove Hospital and the Fountain Hospital probably arose because they were both sited in Tooting Grove. According to information from a former fever nurse, Mrs D. Vera Millard (5 April 2004), who trained at the Grove Hospital (1938–40), 'the gates of the Fountain Hospital were opposite the Grove.'

15 Ayers (1971), p. 274.

16 As a result of the Local Government Board Act, 1871, a new board was set up to supervise the Poor Law and public health; the MAB was, therefore, under the Metropolitan Poor Act, 1867, subject to its control.

17 Ayers (1971), p. 149.

18 Data from English Heritage (10 October 2003) and *The Builder*, 4 November 1893: 342–43.

19 Annual Report, MAB, 1893, properly titled Metropolitan Asylums Board, Annual Report 1893 of the Statistical Committee and the Medical Superintendents of the Infectious Hospitals and Imbecile Asylums, also of the Ambulance and Training Ship 'Exmouth' Committees (Eighth year of Issue), pp. 74–75. The annual reports 1894–96 give Dr C. E. Matthews as Medical Superintendent of the Fountain.

20 Goffman (1991[1961]), p. 16

21 Royal London Hospital Archives (RLHA) LH/N/1/5, London Hospital register of probationers no. 5, 1895–96. This record states the facts as Edith appeared in training at the London. Between September 1896 and February 1898, she was posted late forty-six times. Being late for breakfast could indicate that a nurse had fallen ill. Miss Lückes had been accused in 1890 of overworking her nurses and began to note lateness thereafter.

22 LMA Photographic Library, 26.15 FOU. The following words were written by a member of staff on the back of this photograph, 'Edith Cavell's application to join the staff of Fountain's [sic] Fever Hospital'.

23 RLHA LH/N/1/5. London Hospital register of probationers no. 5, 1895–96.

24 Clark-Kennedy (1965), pp. 26–27.

25 Parker and Collins (1998), p. 65.

26 RLHA LH/N/1/5. London Hospital register of probationers no. 5, 1895–96.

27 RLHA LH/N/7/7/30. Reference for Edith Cavell by the Matron of the Fountain Hospital, Lower Tooting, London, dated 25 April 1896.

28 RLHA LH/N/7/7/30. Reference for Edith Cavell by Mrs Roberts, Norfolk, dated 25 April 1896.

29 *Burdett's Hospitals and Charities, 1899*. This yearbook gives the following information about the Fountain: Beds 402; Matron, Miss K. L. Burleigh; 1 Assistant Matron; 1 Night Superintendent; 18 Charge Nurses; Assistant Nurses: 35 Class I; 42 Class II.

30 Annual Report, MAB, 1895, Fountain Hospital section, p. 73.

31 The diphtheria bacillus was first discovered by Klebs in 1883 and isolated by Löffler in 1884. Ayers (1971), pp. 86, 98.
32 Hardy (1993), p. 103.
33 Annual Report, MAB, 1895, p. 71.
34 Ayers (1971), p. 286.
35 Hardy (1993), pp. 64, 74.
36 Ibid., pp. 74, 76.
37 Ibid., p. 67.
38 Ibid., pp. 151–52.
39 Annual Report, MAB, 1896, Fountain Hospital section, pp. 57–59. By 1896, the MAB had two large convalescent hospitals, the Northern at Winchmore Hill (1887) and the Southern (Upper) at Dartford, Kent (1890). See Ayers (1971), pp. 81, 274.
40 RLHA LH/N/1/5, London Hospital register of probationers, no. 5, 1895–96. This register does not specify where Edith nursed infectious cases, other than at Maidstone.
41 Parker and Collins (1998), pp. 22–23.
42 RLHA LH/N/5/4 London Hospital Private Nursing Institution register of nurses No. 4, 1898–1900.
43 Clark-Kennedy (1965), pp. 42–57.
44 *BJN*, 23 October 1915: 328.
45 S. Kirby (2002) 'Reciprocal Rewards: British Poor Law Nursing and the Campaign for State Registration', *International History of Nursing Journal*, 17(2): 8. See also Ayers (1971), p.149, note 1, for other data regarding infirmaries and training schools.
46 *BJN*, 6 November 1915: 381.
47 Engels (1969[1845]), p. 314.
48 M. Dean and G. Bolton (1980) 'The Administration of Poverty and the Development of Nursing Practice in Nineteenth Century England', in Davies (1980), p. 96.
49 Many TB patients were also admitted to the Brompton, Royal Chest and London Chest hospitals.
50 RLHA LH/N/7/7/3 Letter from Edith Cavell to Eva Lückes, dated 7 October 1904. This Hospital opened in 1869 as the National Cottage Hospital for Consumption and Diseases of the Chest, later known as the Royal National Hospital for Consumption and Diseases of the Chest. It closed in 1964. Laidlaw (1990), p. 7.
51 Ryder (1975), pp. 228–29.
52 *BJN*, September 1926: 195. I was assured that this service still took place when I saw the memorial in 1992.

# 7  Two influential fever nurses

Of the 'real' nurses there are . . . two varieties, those whose interests are mainly clinical, who like the actual treatment of disease; and others who have a latent hankering after administrative work, and will probably ultimately become Matrons. To both of these the fever hospital has something to offer.

Dr A. Knyvett Gordon (1907)[1]

## Introduction

Thousands of young women worked and trained in isolation (fever) hospitals in the late nineteenth and twentieth centuries, so it seems invidious to select just two from those who decided to spend virtually their whole career in fever nursing. Susan Villiers (1863–1945) and Harriet Cassells (b. 1926) were chosen as they epitomise the essence of this speciality from management and clinical perspectives, respectively. These accounts of their lives confirm primary source material cited previously and enhance the overall picture of fever nursing. They lived in different periods when the norms and expectations of society to the admission of patients to hospital and to women in nursing, especially married women working outside the home, were very different. Their backgrounds were different and yet, despite these variations, there were similarities. Both undertook general nurse training, but forsook it in favour of fever nursing in large city hospitals and both showed a wider sense of duty than was strictly necessary through their professional activities, even after retirement. However, there is no intention to present hagiographical or triumphalist narratives, nor to make direct comparisons – they stand as individuals. Nevertheless, they did not exist alone, divorced from their context. The twentieth century, the main period considered here, encompassed major political, social and economic changes. As some of these were relevant to them personally and to working practices in fever nursing, they are included to further understanding of their lives.

Their biographies rely on a variety of mainly primary and some secondary sources. Susan Villiers is solely dependent on impersonal documentary evidence based on a much smaller piece.[2] It is necessarily more objective than that of Harriet Cassells, one of the 127 fever nurses who responded to requests for information about fever nursing for a research project begun in 1994–95 and published in 1998[3], but which then continued to 2002. Evidence from her questionnaire, certificates, training schedules, letters, photographs and a citation from the Royal College of Nursing in 1985, plus the great benefit of being able to converse with her to obtain more details, form the basis of her more personal biography. It also demonstrates the wisdom of getting first-hand accounts of nursing care from nurses before it is too late.

## Susan Alice Villiers (1863–1945)

### Background

Susan Villiers was one of the most eminent fever nurses of her generation, yet, perhaps, surprisingly she was not formally fever nurse trained, as no such nationally recognised course existed in 1892, when she began her general nurse training course. Despite this, she rose to the height of her profession to become Matron, successively, to three large isolation hospitals in early-twentieth-century London. Susan took a major part in the setting up of a national fever nurse training course from 1908, and was the fever nurse representative of the new General Nursing Council for England and Wales from 1920 to 1937. She was also a contemporary and supporter of Mrs Bedford Fenwick, née Ethel Gordon Manson (1857–1947), Matron of St Bartholomew's Hospital, London (Bart's), 1881–87, originator of the movement for the state registration of nurses.

Susan was born on 6 September 1863, at Chase Vale, Edmonton, Middlesex, the eighth of nine children born to Mary Anne (1825–99) and John Fitzpatrick Villiers (*c.*1816–74). Both her father and paternal grandfather were barristers of law at Gray's Inn and eventually her brother, Richard John (1850–1913), became an attorney and a solicitor. Little is known of Susan's youth. Census returns show that the family moved frequently; in 1871 they lived at Waterfall Farm, East Barnet; in 1881 they were in Islington, but by 1891 they were back in Edmonton, living at Highfield House. They also reveal that at least one or two indoor servants were employed, as was the custom in large middle-class families. Susan was privately educated and appears to have lived at home until she was 28 years old. As a spinster daughter, she would probably have shared in the household management with her mother. Such families rarely sent their sick into hospitals; they were nursed at home by family, their own servants, or private nurses.

In the nineteenth century, the role of a middle-class mother was often that of a chatelaine (or housekeeper), which included supervision of the household and the sick. On a much larger scale, these were the main duties of a hospital matron then. This may have explained Susan's initial interest in nursing. As her father had died intestate in 1874 when she was only 11 years old, leaving less than £300,[4] and it seemed she was unlikely to marry, her mind could have turned to nursing, which offered accommodation as well as training with a small salary. By the 1890s, nursing was becoming a respectable profession and, therefore, more acceptable in the social circles in which she moved.

## General nurse training, 1892–95

On 1 May 1892, Susan began a three-year course of general nurse training as a 'special probationer' at Bart's. The probationer system started there in 1877 to supply the hospital with trained nurses of its own; they were from a wide range of backgrounds. In 1884, the Matron, Miss Manson, introduced a distinction. 'Ladies desirous of acquiring some practical knowledge of nursing could become "special probationers", for a period of three months, on payment of a fee. The intention was to attract ladies of a superior class.'[5]

Social class, although divisive, was very important then; nurses, like other people, knew, or were expected to know, their place. Strict hierarchies pertained in all spheres, including large households, the army and nursing. Susan's initial interest in hospital nursing, as opposed to care in a domestic setting, increased after her initial time as a special probationer and she became an ordinary probationer in November 1892 to improve her experience. Isla Stewart had succeeded Miss Manson as Matron following her marriage to Dr Bedford Fenwick in 1887. Susan was awarded her hospital certificate of efficiency in April 1895 and was appointed staff nurse in May. She resigned in March 1896, having been appointed Night Superintendent at the MAB South Eastern Fever Hospital, New Cross, South London. In her reference, Miss Stewart wrote:

> St Bartholomew's Hospital, London, E C,
> 5th March 1897 [*sic*]
>
> Miss Susan Villiers entered the service of the Hospital in May 1892 after three years service, and having passed two examinations, she was awarded a Certificate of efficiency, she remained in the service of the Hospital until March 1896.
>
> During that time she worked in Medical, Surgical, Diphtheria and Ophthalmic Wards.
>
> I found Miss Villiers a most capable and conscientious nurse. Intelligent kind and tactful in her dealings with her patients, very loyal to her superiors in Office and pleasant and considerate to her fellow nurses.
>
> Isla Stewart
> Matron and Supt of nurses[6]

## Rationale for a career in fever nursing

It is important to consider the reasons why Susan, a certificated general nurse, chose to work in a fever hospital. As explained in Chapter 2, the creation of most fever and smallpox hospitals was relatively slow in the nineteenth century, but in larger cities, such as London, where the population escalated in the nineteenth century, the authorities felt obliged to implement measures in order to protect the public health. The population in London reached 1 million in 1811, over 2 million in 1851 and passed 3 million in the 1860s. By the 1880s it was over 4 million.[7]

As a result of the Metropolitan Poor Act, 1867, the first state system of fever, smallpox and mental hospitals was set up in London, initially for the poor. Between 1870 and 1899, the new MAB established nine large permanent fever hospitals and one temporary one, at different points of the compass surrounding London, and between 1887 and 1902 added three convalescent fever hospitals, plus two others which could be used for either fever or smallpox patients, and two hospitals specifically for smallpox patients.[8] The emphasis initially was primarily to prevent the spread of, often fatal, infectious diseases within the metropolis, as much as to treat the individual. In 1867 Florence Nightingale had suggested that the planned new hospitals should be used to train nurses as well as for medical instruction.[9] However, fever nurse training in MAB hospitals had not begun when Susan took up her first post with this organisation in 1896. Most of the nursing then was carried out by untrained female assistant nurses, but the attrition rate was relatively high. The demand for them to staff these new hospitals may have been great, but even more so was the need for trained fever nurse leaders.

## Posts with the Metropolitan Asylums Board

Towards the end of the nineteenth century, some large voluntary general hospitals and a few city fever hospitals in Britain had already begun to appoint mainly middle-class, trained nurses as matrons instead of housekeepers. Isla Stewart had been employed by the MAB from 1885 to 1887 as matron of a major smallpox camp on the Thames' estuary at Darenth, Dartford, Kent and at the Eastern Fever Hospital, Homerton Grove, London. She considered that her employment with the Board was the best possible school for matrons.[10] Since its inception, it had followed a system of rotation of legally qualified doctors and certificated nurses between its hospitals, to widen their experience and to enable the system to benefit as they took more senior posts. As Table 7.1 shows, Susan Villiers became involved in this process. She held responsible posts in five large MAB fever hospitals, most of them newly established.

Isla Stewart is known to have kept in touch with some of her ex-probationers. On 6 May 1901, she wrote to Susan congratulating her on her new appointment at the Fountain. 'I am exceedingly glad it has gone to one of us and I hope you will like it and be very happy there. Dr Matthews seems to be a pleasant Superintendent to work with'. She hoped that Susan would come and see her some day when she was in town, 'you will find the Fountain more getatable than the Brook'.[11] The term 'us' was probably a reference to those in the pro-registration of nurses' faction, headed by Mrs Fenwick. Susan's

*Table 7.1* Susan Villiers' career pathway in MAB fever hospitals, 1896–1927, with their opening dates

| | | |
|---|---|---|
| South Eastern (1877) | Night Superintendent | 1896–99 |
| Brook (1896) | Assistant Matron | 1899–1901 |
| Fountain (1893) | Matron | 1901–10 |
| Park (1897) | Matron | 1910–13 |
| South Western (1871) | Matron | 1913–27 |

Source: G. M. Ayers (1971) *England's First State Hospitals 1867–1930*, London: Wellcome Institute of the History of Medicine, pp. 97, 274; London Metropolitan Archives, Metropolitan Asylums Board Board Minutes; letter, dated 6 May 1901, from Isla Stewart to Susan Villiers on her appointment as Matron of the Fountain Hospital, King's College London Archives

three years as Night Superintendent at the South Eastern Hospital must have been quite a learning experience. Although it is known that she nursed patients with diphtheria and, probably, other infectious diseases at Bart's, it is unlikely that she would have been exposed to them on such a major scale. In fact, it was the experience she gained at the South Eastern which was cited later in order for her to register as a fever nurse with the GNC for England and Wales.[12]

The MAB is known to have participated in joint schemes of training between its Western Fever Hospital and Guy's Hospital in 1901,[13] and, as was seen in Chapter 2, between Irish general and children's hospitals and the North Western Hospital. Knowledge of this may have persuaded Susan towards the benefits of joint schemes.[14] By the late nineteenth century, some large, and a few small, fever hospitals had already begun their own specific fever nurse courses and issued certificates to this effect, but there was no standardisation in length, content or clinical experience anywhere in Britain.

The most knowledgeable people were the matrons and medical superintendents of large fever hospitals, and it was they who formed the dominant nucleus of the Fever Nurses' Association, established in 1908, described fully in Chapter 2. Urged on by Mrs Fenwick, as editor of her own publication the *British Journal of Nursing*, the FNA aimed to provide a uniform system of training. Susan Villiers, by then Matron of the Fountain Hospital, was one of ten MAB matrons and assistant matrons appointed to their first governing body in June 1908 (see Appendix 2). She was directly involved in the decision to approve large hospitals with a resident medical officer, for a two-year course for women without previous experience and a one-year course for general nurses who had trained at a hospital of which the FNA approved. In effect, these decisions meant that young women, who were purportedly 'trained' at small rural hospitals without a resident doctor, could gain no remission in the length of their general nurse course, unlike FNA trained nurses, who benefited from a one-year remission. The FNA syllabus was approved for use in MAB fever hospitals in July 1909.[15] Susan Villiers, as Matron, successively, of three such institutions, was in an ideal position to monitor the progress of courses and, with the Medical Superintendent, suggest any modifications.

## State registration and further responsibilities

The three new GNCs set up under the Nurses (Registration) Acts, 1919, for England and Wales, Scotland and Ireland were left to decide the various parts of the register that were needed by the profession from their perspective. For example, the GNC for England and Wales concluded that the general part was to be the main register; other branches, including fever nursing, and the one for male nurses, were to be supplementary registers.[16] Nurses of Susan Villiers' generation were proud of their training hospitals and the certificates they issued, but large numbers of them saw the wisdom of being included in the new registers which gave them, for the first time, a qualification recognised by the state.

Susan was entitled to an entry in the General Register by virtue of her training and certificate from Bart's (1892–95). The date of her registration as a general nurse was 30 September 1921. She was the seventh entry and her permanent address was given as the South Western Hospital, Landor Road, London SW9. Mrs Fenwick had the honour of being the first nurse recorded in what was clearly soon seen by the general public and a major part of the profession as the most prestigious register.[17] Susan's name was also recorded in the Supplementary Register of Fever Nurses. The date of her registration was 17 March 1922; her address was the same and she was the sixtieth entry. According to this Fever Register she was 'trained 1896–99',[18] although she was actually in employment at the South Eastern Hospital then as Night Superintendent, not a probationer. Susan Villiers was now allowed to add the initials SRN, RFN after her name.

In 1920, she became the fever nurse representative to the Caretaker GNC for England and Wales and she continued in that capacity in the elected council from 1923 to 1937. Susan was one of sixteen nurse members of this new GNC. At that time she was Matron of the South Western Hospital, treasurer and vice-president of the Matrons' Council of Great Britain and Ireland and a member of the executive and council of the Royal British Nurses' Association, member of the executive of the National Union of Trained Nurses and delegate of the Central Committee. Her genuine belief in the integration of fever and general nurse training was clearly stated in a paper she gave on reciprocal training at an Informal Conference on the Supplementary Registers, held at the Royal Society of Medicine on 28 April 1921.[19] Nevertheless, these two areas of nursing remained separate entities, with different qualifications, but it was mainly on Susan's advice that the GNC adopted the tried and tested FNA scheme of training, virtually unchanged, in 1923.

It is clear from MAB minutes that Susan had another professional role: she was an approved examiner for examinations taken by nurses at their fever hospitals. At a meeting on 9 February 1924, the MAB, having taken advice from the Ministry of Health, approved the payment of examiners' fees for the previous October examinations at the rate of £42 for the Principal

Examiner, Dr F. Foord Caiger, Chief Medical Officer infectious hospitals service and Dr Matthews, Medical Superintendent, Northern Hospital, and £21 each to two matrons, Miss S. Villiers (South Western Fever Hospital) and Miss N. Butler (Southern Convalescent Fever Hospital).[20]

## Responsibilities in retirement, and travel to Europe, Canada and United States

Susan had been off duty through illness on at least two occasions in 1922 and 1924 due, probably, to cardiac asthma from which she was known to suffer.[21] Having already taken on other professional interests, she decided to retire at the age of 63 years. At a MAB meeting on 17 March 1927, reference was made to the fact that she would retire on superannuation at the end of March. The chairman that day, Mr West, briefly referred to Miss Villiers' long and meritorious service and expressed the hope that she would enjoy good health for many years to come in her retirement.[22]

Having lived in hospital accommodation for thirty-five years, she was at last free to live again in the community. She moved to Stevenage, Hertfordshire, where some of her siblings had settled and was appointed a county magistrate for Stevenage Petty Sessional Division.[23] Her brother, Francis John (1851–1925), had been a Justice of the Peace (JP) there as were her sisters, Fanny (1847–1932) and Annie (1861–1930). Women could not become JPs until 1919, when, following the Representation of the People Act, 1918, they were given the vote, if they were over 30 years of age, ratepayers or wives of ratepayers; the Villiers sisters were probably pioneers in that district.[24] Susan had also been an elected councillor of the British College of Nurses since its inception in 1926.[25] It was founded by Mrs Fenwick as an educational body with a postgraduate college to provide nurses with membership and fellowship by examination. Mrs Fenwick, and colleagues like Susan who supported her, intended that the BCN would provide nurses who wanted it, with professional self-government and with the opportunity of professional development.[26] It was very controversial in its time as it was set up in opposition to the College of Nursing established in 1916 (RCN in 1939), which intended to promote a general standard of training for nurses.

The first vice-president of the BCN was Margaret Breay, one of the close circle of friends and colleagues of Mrs Fenwick and Susan.[27] Under the dominant leadership of Mrs Fenwick, Susan became involved with other issues, for example, she was the representative for the Matrons' Council of Great Britain and Ireland on the National Council of Women of Great Britain.[28] On 26 February 1927, Susan was also named as a vice-president of the BCN, and she agreed to attend a meeting of the National Union of Societies for Equal Citizenship at the Central Hall, Westminster, on 3 March to represent the BCN in support of equal suffrage.[29] Although the Representation of the People Act, 1918, had given the vote to men over 21 years and to women over 30, it did not apply to women over 21 years (then the age of majority), a blatant disregard of equal rights. Susan was honoured with one of the first BCN fellowships in 1927, awarded for her contribution to the advancement of professional nurses. She is shown in a photograph taken at the full graduation ceremony on 27 April 1927 in the robes of a Member of Council, which she wore with dignity and pleasure (Figure 7.1).[30] She appears to be a serene, lady-like person, with a charming manner, attributes confirmed in her Bart's references. Although she retired from the GNC in 1937, she remained a member of the BCN.

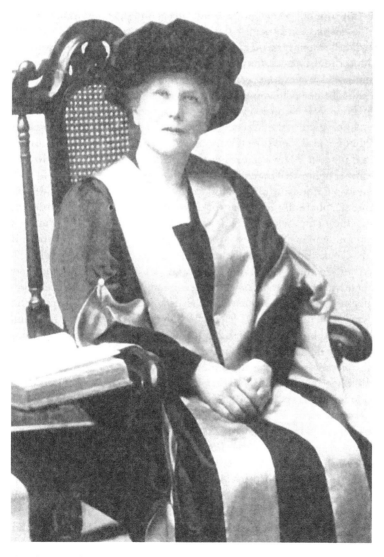

*Figure 7.1* Susan Villiers in her robes as a Member of Council of the British College of Nurses, 1927. King's College London Archives

It is clear that Susan was still professionally active in Britain and abroad in retirement. She participated fully in the GNC and BCN meetings and continued to attend nursing conferences, such as the International Nursing Conference convened by the International Council of Nurses (ICN) at Geneva in 1927.[31] In so doing, she maintained a congenial social circle. Documents, including personal correspondence to Margaret Breay, reveal her sense of humour. On 28 June 1929, she left Southampton on the Cunard liner, *Alaunia*, bound for the Congress of the ICN in Montreal, Canada. Thomas Cook, the official travel agents for the Congress, declared it was 'an ideal holiday ship, and worthily upholds the Cunard traditions of a high standard of comfort and service'.[32] Susan, and other British nurses, apparently enjoyed the outward voyage and the Congress, including time spent afterwards in New York, where they found the American nurses just as hospitable in their own homes as the Canadians.[33] However, the return voyage was on a different ship, the *Caronia*, where she and her colleagues 'had very bad cabins with no light or air'. She thought the accommodation was very poor indeed and vowed never to travel by their line again without seeing the cabins, as they varied so enormously. Even though she tipped the steward and stewardess to get a cabin to herself, 'it was a dungeon'.[34] Her professional interests took much of her time, but her Protestant religion still meant a lot to her.

Susan was a Superior of the Guild of St Barnabas, established in 1876 to help nurses spiritually in their work and life; Barnabas is regarded as the patron saint of nurses. She had held office as honorary secretary of the National Council of Nurses of Great Britain and was known as an efficient honorary treasurer of this body, managing to keep it progressively affluent during the Second World War. Susan did not forget her nursing roots at Bart's and she kept in touch with its League of Nurses until September 1942 when her name finally appeared in the lists of League members.[35] She had been living with her niece, Mary Judith Abbott, daughter of her only married sister, Mary Abbott (b. 1853), at her home in Hindhead, Surrey, for some time after the death of her remaining sister, Fanny, in 1932.

Towards the end of the Second World War her health failed further. Her will, dated 22 February 1945, was signed in a shaky hand, in comparison to earlier correspondence seen. She died five weeks later, on 29 March 1945, at the age of 81 years, from a cerebral haemorrhage due to arteriosclerosis. Her niece, who was present at the death, which took place at her home, Little Nutcombe, Portsmouth Road, Hindhead, received the majority of the net value of her estate: £10,646 8s 4d. Two legacies were bequeathed: £500 to Dorothy Margaret Villiers and £100 to her nephew, Edward Flannery Villiers, a captain in the Royal Pay Corps. Susan's relatively wealthy estate was almost certainly derived from siblings' wills, not from nursing. She was buried on 3 April at St Alban's Church, Hindhead, followed by a well-attended requiem mass on 12 April at St Alban's Church, Holborn, London, organised by the Guild of St Barnabas as a celebration of her life's work.

## Conclusion

Susan Villiers was one of the first generation of general nurses to be trained under a professional nurse. Isla Stewart set high standards at Bart's, based on those established by the previous Matron, Miss Manson (later Mrs Bedford Fenwick). Instead of opting for posts in prestigious, large voluntary hospitals, Susan, probably inspired by Miss Stewart's experience with the MAB, decided to work with fever patients and nurses within that organisation. Although professionally and socially less acceptable, she found in fever nursing a specialism in which she could be effective. However, the decision by the FNA to introduce a two-year course for fever nurses in 1908 contributed to its continuation at that length by all three GNCs, for reasons of reciprocity between countries. Certainly, because the Fever Register was a supplementary register and it was the only one which specified two instead of three years' training, it was seen as less prestigious.[36] Had Susan been less reserved, and more assertive, like Mrs Fenwick, fever nursing could perhaps have become more important professionally. Nevertheless, despite setbacks, she contributed greatly to the development of professional fever nursing. Without her influence and support, it is unlikely that Susan would have flourished and reached such fulfilment in her working life and retirement.

In her personal life, she enjoyed the friendship of other nurse leaders, at meetings, international conferences and on visits to their homes. However, like other Victorians who came from large families, she suffered many bereavements, in particular her father when she was only 11 years old, and her siblings who mostly died before her, as she was the eighth of nine children. Her own death merited a brief mention in *The Times*, but it was her long-time friend, Mrs Fenwick, who wrote a full obituary in the *BJN* in April 1945. The piece was headed, 'The death of Miss Susan Alice Villiers, SRN, RFN, FBCN', proudly proclaiming not only the two state registerable qualifications these ladies had strived so hard to achieve, but also the Fellowship of the British College of Nurses, the organisation in which they both strongly believed. Mrs Fenwick summed up her feelings in the following eulogy, 'Thus has passed to rest one of our sincerely loved leaders. As these great leaders pass on succeeding generations of nurses should not fail to study their life's work and realise its inspiration'.[37] Harriet Cassells and her contemporaries were a new generation with different opportunities and challenges, but fighting for improvements in existing practices in fever nursing was still not to prove easy.

## Harriet May Cassells (b. 1926)

### Background

Harriet Cassells (née Thompson), an eminent fever nurse in Northern Ireland, was awarded a fellowship of the Royal College of Nursing (FRCN) in 1985, the highest honour a nurse can receive from the profession. And yet, she would be the first to say that she began as an ordinary fever nurse, typical of the thousands who trained in the first half of twentieth-century Britain. Following qualification as a RFN and SRN in the 1940s, she chose to spend the major part of her career in clinical nursing, at the bedside, with fever patients, despite being urged to move into management or nurse education. In fact, Harriet was the first ward sister to be awarded an RCN fellowship; she believed it was a recognition of her speciality, infectious diseases, not one of the most glamorous branches in nursing. Harriet was once told that fever nursing was the 'cream on the cake of nursing' because in the early days of poultices, stupes (compresses) and other treatments, it was pure nursing; she agreed and felt that it really was due to devoted nursing care that many patients recovered.

## Rationale for a career in fever nursing

Her background and subsequent personal circumstances may help to explain her reasons for entering fever nursing and then, virtually, remaining in it until retirement in 1990. Born at home on 8 September 1926 in Lifford, County Donegal, she was the second of three children born to her Scottish mother, May Thompson (née McLean) and William Thompson. Harriet May was the middle of three sisters, Jean, three years older and Sandra (Margaret Alexandra), three years younger. They spent their childhood in a rural area, on a farm in County Donegal. During their formative years, from the late 1920s to early 1940s, infectious diseases, although declining nationally, were still rife in some areas. Jean contracted poliomyelitis (polio) in 1926 at the age of 3½ years and was in hospital in Dublin for three years with paralysis of both arms and her left leg; her intercostal muscles were also affected. As she grew up, Harriet witnessed at first hand the disabling effects the disease had on her sister.[38]

Their father, who had served in the 36th Ulster Division of the Royal Engineers in the British Army in the First World War, stayed on until 1921. He had intended to work for the Hudson Bay Company in Canada, but because Jean developed polio, he was not accepted, a decision which had a great effect on the whole family. Harriet herself had pertussis (whooping cough) and measles at, respectively, 3 months and 3 years of age. She recalls epidemics still sweeping through schools in her childhood; one boy she knew died from diphtheria.

She attended Ballindrait National School, Miss Young's Public Elementary Junior School (1930–39) and Prior School, Lifford (1939–43), which was a grammar school. Harriet left school in 1943 having achieved the Intermediate Certificate. During the late 1930s, her father, by now in his fifties, who had been with his regiment at the Battle of the Somme on the Western Front in July 1916, suffered the ill effects of being gassed, with bouts of pneumonia and asthma. Harriet said that as there were no antibiotics and because she felt unable to help him, she used to sit up at night with him. She thinks that it was this experience which influenced her to take up nursing.[39]

## Fever nurse training, 1943–45

Harriet's nursing career began on 19 October 1943, at the Purdysburn Fever Hospital, Belfast (Figure 7.2).[40] The contrast between her rural upbringing and life in the capital city of Northern Ireland, famed for its linen trade and shipbuilding, was very great.[41]

She was the youngest in her preliminary training school at 17 years, 1 month, and could have felt homesick, but she was fortunate that her cousin, Beth Porterfield, was in the same set. Most of the seventeen other probationers who started with her were the same age. Unfortunately, Harriet developed psoriasis in PTS, which delayed her first ward placement, but did not prevent her continuing her career. In her set only twelve qualified: six left due to homesickness or simply because they did not like nursing; the Second World War apparently had little effect on this high wastage rate. At

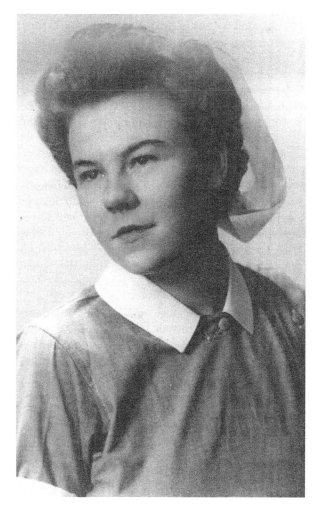

*Figure 7.2* Nurse Harriet Thompson, 1945. Courtesy of Mrs Harriet Cassells

that time, there were three or four intakes of ten to fourteen probationers annually. Purdysburn was a recognised school of nursing, approved by the Joint Nursing and Midwives' Council for Northern Ireland (JNMCNI). It had a resident medical superintendent and about 350 beds with an almost constant influx of patients with a wide range of infectious diseases – good clinical experience for the nurses.

When Harriet was in training, probationers worked a forty-eight-hour week, with four weeks' annual leave, wisely allocated in the summer before the autumn epidemics began. Night duty hours were 8 p.m. to 7.30 a.m. with three nights off duty after thirteen nights. They were paid £2 2s 0d (£2.10) monthly in the first year, rising to £3 3s 0d (£3.15) in the second year, but full board was provided in a spacious, well-run nurses' home as, in other forms of nurse training then, they were all required to be resident until qualification. No men undertook fever nurse training at Purdysburn until after the Second World War; the first two started in 1947, but only one qualified. He was Mr Robert Graham, who had first completed a three-year SRN course at the City Hospital, Belfast and was, therefore, able to undertake the RFN course in one year.[42]

Harriet was able to return home only once a year for holidays as it was 100 miles from Belfast and the journey was time-consuming. However, her friends and her cousin in the same PTS provided some support. She thought she had found her niche in life, although there were some aspects she disliked in training, including cleaning brass, sluicing napkins and the hassle of disinfecting herself whenever she changed wards, before going into town, and sleeping out. Fortunately, some nurse friends and a widow, known to her family, invited her to their homes, which was particularly welcome when she had three nights off duty and could escape strict hospital routines. The most difficult situations she found were when too much responsibility was placed on her as a junior nurse. For example, it was common practice on night duty to be alone in charge of a ward, except for an occasional visit from the night sister; she particularly remembers those who required technically skilled care such as babies with tracheotomies and patients in iron lungs who gave her cause for concern.

Harriet especially liked caring for children, although she nursed patients of all ages and, because it was wartime, British, Belgian and American service personnel; she therefore became experienced in nursing patients of all ages, of different nationalities, some with language difficulties, with a wide range of diseases including:

| | |
|---|---|
| cerebro-spinal fever | primary TB in children |
| chickenpox (varicella) | pulmonary TB in adults |
| diphtheria | salmonella (adults returning from abroad) |
| dysentery | scarlet fever |
| gastro-enteritis in small infants | Steven Johnson syndrome |

| | |
|---|---|
| hepatitis | tonsillitis and quinsy |
| measles | tropical fevers, including malaria |
| meningitis (all types) | typhoid fever |
| poliomyelitis | whooping cough |

Most patients recovered, but some died. When they were gravely ill, strenuous efforts were made to save them. For instance, Harriet recalls nursing patients with typhoid fever before the introduction of chloramphenicol; they required two good nurses, turpentine stupes (medicated compresses) to the abdomen, plenty of fluids and intensive nursing care. Like most fever nurses, the most seriously ill patients made a deep impression on her. A girl from the Auxiliary Territorial Service with typhoid fever who died in 1945 has not been forgotten. According to Harriet, children almost invariably died of tuberculous meningitis by the twenty-first day, until the introduction of streptomycin in the early 1950s. She recalls the first patient to be treated with penicillin in Northern Ireland in *c.*1944–45, a 17-year-old boy who had been bitten by a rat and had developed rat bite fever. The new drug had to be administered three hourly by intramuscular injection; he eventually made a good recovery.[43]

Children with measles were nursed in steam tents. Although steam kettles were particularly hazardous because of their long spouts, which children could grab, they were later found to be more effective than modern humidifiers, as long as great care was taken to protect children from scalds. When wards were cubicalised (1951–52), steam jets from the central heating were placed in special cubicles for patients requiring steam treatment, a facility rarely seen elsewhere. Children with croup or laryngeal diphtheria were intubated (a tube inserted into the larynx). When they were recovering, the medical officer asked them to say, 'Billy Bunter bought a buttered biscuit', to see if they had paralysis of their vocal cords and spoke through their noses. Before being allowed home, patients went through the special procedure carried out in most large and small fever hospitals in a separate discharge block. First, they stripped off their ward clothes, bathed in disinfected water and then donned clean clothes ready for home; they were never allowed back into the ward.

There was a smallpox compound nearby, but, although this disease was covered in the syllabus of training, Harriet did not nurse patients with this disease. During her fever training, some colleagues contracted infectious diseases from their patients; she developed chickenpox which lengthened her training by twelve weeks, as sick leave had to be made up to conform with the statutory two years. Many girls had little or no immunity, especially those from country areas, so they often caught measles. Some probationers became carriers of diphtheria; although, technically, they were not still ill, they had to be isolated, but were allowed to work on that ward. However, during two major polio epidemics, not one nurse contracted the disease.

The 'Schedule of Class and Ward Work for Probationer Nurses' training in Fever Nursing' set out by the JNMCNI shows the great emphasis placed on practical ward work, as opposed to class work, which required fifteen topics to be covered from ward etiquette to verbal reports for medical officers. The seventy-eight different tasks to be achieved in the two years began with 'cleaning' and ended with 'last offices'; all had to be signed by ward sisters to signify competence. The majority of this work was common to those in general nurse training, hence, the three-year course, for those who undertook it, was reduced to two years for fever nurses. Harriet's schedule also shows where she was 'stationed' in training and as a staff nurse. Although it was not the norm in many isolation hospitals then, according to her schedule, the first four weeks were spent in PTS.[44] During this time, the new probationers had their Schick and Dick tests for diphtheria and scarlet fever and, if necessary, were immunised. They were also protected with a typhoid vaccine. Although they were given a Mantoux test for tuberculosis, no vaccine was available at that time to protect them against the disease.

During her training, Harriet rotated between the diphtheria, scarlatina, isolation, measles and typhoid wards at irregular intervals according to service requirements, not apparently to benefit her educationally. Lectures, plus notes, were given by Miss Adams the Sister Tutor, Dr Kane, the Medical Superintendent, other doctors and, occasionally, the Matron, Miss Anne C. Cameron. The set also had 'talks' from the man responsible for fumigating patients' clothing, mattresses and pillows, and during a visit to the pathology laboratory. Like her colleagues, she also attended post-mortems. Probationers at Purdysburn had some textbooks: anatomy and physiology (Evelyn Pearce), nursing (Pugh) and one on hygiene in order to prepare for the first and second part of the state preliminary examinations, plus a copy of Dr Kane's lecture notes.

## Registered fever nurse and general training, 1947–49

Harriet had completed her training by early 1945, but was not permitted to take the final examination for fever nurses until February 1946, when she had made up sick leave. During her training, the Matron of Purdysburn Fever Hospital, Miss Cameron, who had been in post since February 1934, died in January 1945, after a long illness due to cancer. A fund was set up in her memory to award prizes to the best all-round nurse of the year. Harriet was the first recipient of this very coveted award in October 1946.[45] Her prize was to be a book, which had to be approved by the committee. Although she wanted a history of nursing, there was not one available and she eventually chose a history of medicine, which received the necessary authorisation.[46] Her RFN certificate for the Supplementary Part of the Register was not issued by the JNMCNI until 22 October 1947, the age of 21 years being the earliest allowed for registration (see Appendix 4.8). By then, Harriet was already involved in her general nurse training at the Belfast City Hospital, which was completed in just over two years in 1949. In fact, she had applied earlier to do her training to become a SRN at St Mary's Hospital,

Paddington, in London, but was informed that they 'had enough Irish nurses'. Fortunately, this was not really a setback as she enjoyed her time at the City Hospital. Following this, she gained experience as a staff nurse in theatres until 1950, when she returned to her fever training hospital, now known as the Northern Ireland Fever Hospital, as a ward sister.

## Ward sister, marriage and a career break

In the early 1950s, student nurses from the Royal Belfast Hospital for Sick Children and the Royal Victoria Hospital, Belfast, did a six to eight weeks' placement. In the late 1960s, female and male pupil nurses from Purdysburn Mental Hospital and Forester Green Hospital, a former TB sanatorium, converted to a hospital for neurology and care of elderly people, attended for children's training when it became an enrolled nurse training school. Medical students from Queen's University, Belfast, attended lectures given by Dr Kane, and did ward rounds with him, when they were shown any unusual rashes and other significant features of infectious diseases. GPs taking their Public Health Certificate also attended lectures and ward rounds.

Harriet's first post as a ward sister was, therefore, in a centre of excellence. She felt ready for the responsibility, but did not always find management easy. For instance, having worked in theatres, she wanted to introduce more modern aseptic techniques and make changes in sterilisation methods, but they were achieved only after a battle. Further struggles ensued as she fought for the rights and welfare of student and, later, pupil nurses. During the early 1950s, Harriet was 'involved with research into the treatment of tuberculous meningitis when streptomycin first came on the scene'.[47] However, before she left the fever hospital, for her general training, she had met Joseph Cassells, known as Joe, who had served in the Second World War and had been at Dunkirk. He began work at Purdysburn in 1946 as a hospital engineer. Initially, his work included driving one of the three special green Humber fever ambulances kept at the hospital, and he was the last driver to use one in 1947. Joe, who worked in this large fever hospital until his retirement in 1976, was highly regarded by all the staff.

Harriet and Joe's marriage took place at McCrocken Presbyterian Church, Belfast on 13 June 1951. Harriet was the first married sister at the Northern Ireland Fever Hospital (previously Purdysburn); she paved the way for others. She remained in post until 1956. Three sons were born: Andrew (28 February 1957), John (6 December 1958) and Joseph (10 December 1961). She found fever nursing to be a good foundation for motherhood. While rearing her family she was often called in by neighbours to diagnose various rashes and advise on infectious diseases. During the time when she had only two sons, her neighbour's children had mumps. Harriet, wearing a white coat, went in to see them only at night but, nevertheless, she contracted the disease, as did Andrew and John. She was not infallible.

## Resumption of career and open visiting

In 1964 she resumed her career, after an eight-year break, by working part-time in the field of radiotherapy and cancer care at the new centre opened at one end of the Northern Ireland Fever Hospital in 1952. From 1969 to 1990, when she retired, Harriet worked full-time at this hospital (Belvoir Park Hospital from 1975) as a fever ward sister and, as her experience grew, acted in an advisory capacity to other hospitals. She undertook a number of courses to remain up-to-date and was seconded to Coppetts Wood Isolation Hospital, in north London, to learn more about smallpox and other serious, mostly tropical, infections including the use of an isolator for green monkey disease. Her ambition was to be clinical nurse specialist in infection control, a relatively new role for senior nurses, but there was not an opening at that time. Having worked as a part-time staff nurse in the radiotherapy unit for five years (1964–69), where open visiting was allowed, and having seen similar practices at other hospitals, Harriet wanted to introduce bedside visiting of parents for children with infectious diseases in her ward. She reasoned that if students, chaplains and others on hospital business could visit the ward with no apparent ill effect, parents, who had even more valid reasons, should also be permitted. Her logic may have been based on her empathy with parents, as at that time she had a young family herself. She had already carried out a pilot scheme with parents of children with tuberculous meningitis, who were not then infectious. However, allowing visitors for some but not all children proved controversial, so she decided to introduce open visiting in 1974.

It proved to be a battle and she was told that, were there to be any cross-infection she would be held responsible. Harriet and the other qualified nurses instructed parents very carefully in order to avoid this. The decision was not necessarily popular with all the staff. In many ways it transferred the onus of care from nursing staff back to parents, but in so doing, took away much of the pleasure nurses had derived in caring for children, who they sometimes regarded, possessively, as their own. This was a problem which had been highlighted in the inquiry, *The Welfare of Children in Hospital*, chaired by Sir Harry Platt. In The Platt Report, published in 1959, the recommendations included meeting the mental and emotional needs of children by encouraging the parents to visit at all times, helping with the nursing and allowing children to bring in and keep their favourite toys. 'Above all, nurses had to learn to understand their own emotional attitudes to children and their own natural desire to gain a child's affection'. Seemingly, child psychology now overrode nurse training where the first consideration was hygiene and the avoidance of infection. 'Children should only be admitted to hospital as a last resort, nursed in special units under the supervision of a sick children's nurse and a paediatrician'.[48] Employment of sick children's nurses proved difficult, as they seldom stayed long in the fever hospital. Although the Platt Report had made these recommendations in 1959, they had not been implemented at the Belvoir Park Hospital. It is clear that managers had distinct reservations. It took Harriet to solve the visiting problem.

## Fellowship of the Royal College of Nursing

Harriet was undoubtedly a capable lady with attributes and experience which were later recognised nationally. In 1985 she became a Fellow of the Royal College of Nursing, the citation for which gives the justification for this prestigious award. It is quoted verbatim.

Harriet May Cassells
elected
Fellow of the Royal College of Nursing

Harriet May Cassells has been nursing since 1943 and has throughout her career stayed, by choice, in the clinical field despite on many occasions having been invited to enter higher management or teaching grades. As a result, the profession in Northern Ireland has benefited from her dedication to clinical nursing and from her innovation in the clinical setting in which she takes a particular interest in teaching at ward level.

Harriet Cassells qualified in 1946 as a Registered Fever Nurse, and as a State Registered Nurse in 1949. Since 1969, she has been a Nursing Sister at the Belvoir Park Hospital in Belfast and before that held various staff appointments in the Province. During this time, Harriet Cassells has made infection control one of her specialities, and in 1951 she introduced new aseptic techniques and modern methods of sterilization while working as a Sister in the Northern Ireland Fever Hospital. She has also taken a special interest in services for children and parents at ward level and in 1974 she introduced the procedure of allowing parents into infectious areas and instructing them in the prevention of infection by involving them, more closely in the care of their children. Previous to this, parents had not been allowed direct contact with their children who were being barrier nursed. In furthering her clinical interest, Harriet Cassells has undertaken, and continues to undertake, clinically-based research and she is at present collaborating with a medical team researching pertussis in Northern Ireland.

Harriet Cassells' dream has always been to see the introduction of the clinical nurse specialist, for which her own career has served as a role model. She has maintained an interest in nursing education at the patient level and improving the ward learning environment for student nurses. She is currently engaged in curriculum planning for a post-registration course on infectious diseases which it is hoped will be implemented in the near future. She also lectures at the Queen's University in Belfast on the subject of infectious disease control, as well as maintaining an active teaching presence within her own hospital to student nurses and other staff.

For almost 40 years Harriet Cassells' dedication to the high standards of care for her patients and to an innovative approach to her own clinical practice has benefited not only her own development as a clinical specialist in infection control nursing but her nursing colleagues and student nurses as well. The Council has great pleasure, therefore, in conferring on Harriet May Cassells Fellowship of the Royal College of Nursing.[49]

The special ceremony was convened for the first time as an integral part of the RCN Annual Congress, held that year in April 1985 in Bournemouth. Sheila Quinn, the RCN president, explained that it was a deliberate action in order that Fellows became part of RCN life. The award comprises a special gold coloured medallion with an enlarged RCN crest, a certificate and the formal citation. The ceremony and special lunch afterwards was attended by Neil Kinnock, then leader of the opposition party. Three other eminent nurses also received fellowships at the ceremony. Baroness Cox of Queensbury received her award for the advancement of nursing and health issues in the House of Lords and elsewhere. Trevor Clay was chosen for his pioneering work in psychiatry, in developing a professional advisory machinery and his efforts to extend participation to all nurses. His long years of activity within the RCN and his international horizons were also mentioned. Allan Pearson's name is synonymous with the Burford Development Unit, where he initiated intriguing developments in expanding the nurse's role; this innovatory work earned him his fellowship. Speaking on behalf of her 'fellow Fellows', Baroness Cox said it was the greatest honour they could have, or ever will have. Nursing was their first love and she believed they would go on promoting the interests of nursing in all their spheres of work.[50]

The award of the FRCN was sufficiently newsworthy for an Irish national newspaper, the *Belfast Telegraph*, to put Harriet's photograph and an article about her on its front page. It mentioned that she was the second nurse in Northern Ireland to be so honoured by the RCN, the first being Kathleen Robb OBE, in 1977, a former district administrative nursing officer of the north and west Belfast district executive team. Harriet said she felt humble and extremely honoured to receive the FRCN, especially as it was the first time it had gone to anyone of her grade in a clinical post.[51]

## Retirement

Twelve years after the award ceremony in Bournemouth and seven years after her retirement, Harriet's husband, Joe, died on 5 August 1997, coincidentally the same day that Belvoir Park Hospital closed. Her middle son, John, a gardener, gave Harriet much support at that time, and he continues to live with her. Fortunately, she has a close family and many friends. She enjoys seeing her other two sons and their wives, and her granddaughter, Louise (18 years) who is currently at the University of Glasgow.[52]

Harriet now spends some of her time learning to swim, gardening and walking with rambling groups. Regrettably, she became ill in 1999 as she developed bronchiectasis, she believes, probably, due to nursing children with pneumonia; her weight dropped from 11 to 7 stone and she was in hospital for four weeks. There was no confirmed diagnosis. Since then, she has made a gradual recovery and is now active in various groups, including, the local Women's Institute and church affairs. She keeps in touch with her professional interests through membership of the Northern Ireland RCN History of Nursing Society. She is also president of the local RCN branch and attends functions, such as fellowship dinners (Figure 7.3) and Nurse of the Year awards where she sees former colleagues and friends, including Kathleen Robb, OBE, FRCN. Harriet is also secretary of the local Health Service Retirement Association. Holidays are sometimes taken through the Holiday Fellowship or with her family. On a daily basis, she enjoys walking her dog with a friend from her fever nurse probationer days, who was two sets below her. As Harriet remarked earlier, 'Fever nurse training brought companionship and long-lasting friendships'. In 2003 she pointed out how much her training hospital meant to her.

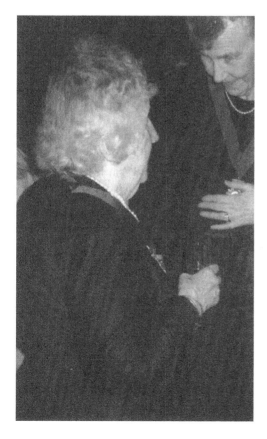

*Figure 7.3* Virginia Henderson FRCN (left) with Harriet Cassells FRCN at the RCN Fellows' dinner, 1988. Courtesy of Miss Kathleen Robb, OBE, FRCN

When my husband and I were ill, friends from Belvoir Park Hospital were wonderful, and still are, especially the younger sisters who come to see me and take me to hospital appointments. I call them my daughters too. I enjoyed my life as a fever nurse and was fortunate to be involved in so many ways. It was particularly gratifying, when nursing meningitis (one of my specialities). The patient was so very ill, but because of nursing intervention recovered, and when small babies were at death's door with pertussis, and because again of the constant observation and attention recovered, entirely due to nurses.[53]

It is clear that Harriet's first love was fever nursing, not superseded until she married. She forged the way for others by continuing to work until she had a family, and typical of her generation, resumed her career on a part-time basis for a few years to fit in with family needs. This clearly did not prevent her achieving national recognition from her profession. Her life, like others, has not been without problems, of which she seems to have made light. Her rejection at a London teaching hospital was just one example. Harriet feels that present-day nurses have such wonderful opportunities. 'We certainly didn't get much encouragement, we had to fight for every change we wanted to make'.[54] It seems that each generation of nurses, whatever their speciality, has to undergo trials and tribulations in order to achieve improvements in patient care. Harriet's career shows that it is possible.

## Conclusion

This chapter covered the major part of the lives of Susan Villiers and Harriet Cassells. In Susan's lifetime, inequalities were seen in the lack of female emancipation and struggles to achieve state registration for fever nurses, both of which she saw achieved. Harriet was faced with different problems. First, the legacy of the First World War, with her father's illness, although it almost certainly led to her taking up a career in nursing. Second, what would now be termed 'racism' in the remark that the hospital had 'enough Irish nurses', which might have prevented her broadening her nursing experience in London, but did not put her off her goal of becoming a state registered nurse. However, she benefited particularly from changing attitudes in society to married women working outside the home after the Second World War.

Whereas Susan chose to remain in senior nurse management posts in which she functioned effectively, and in retirement continued to work for the common good of the profession, Harriet resisted pressure to go into nurse management or education permanently, choosing instead to provide and supervise the proper care of the patient. The RCN citation (1985) describes succinctly the different ways in which she was able to expand her role as a carer. For instance, in services to parents by encouraging and showing them, how to care for their children with infectious diseases, in research and teaching at university level and at the bedside. Harriet was able to continue her career despite being married, whereas Susan's success in nurse management in the early twentieth century was almost certainly dependent on her maintaining her status as a single woman. No evidence of the same discriminatory criteria has been found about men who took up different branches of nursing including fever nursing; single or married, it was not an issue. Research has shown that Susan and Harriet were both positive forces in their chosen speciality. They strove, with their colleagues, to adapt to changes demanded of them, and for improvements they wanted to make for the ultimate benefit of patient care.

## Notes and references*

1 A. K. Gordon (1907) 'The Position of the Isolation Hospital in the Training of a Nurse', *BJN*, 26 January: 63.
2 This was commissioned by the Oxford University Press as one of 50,0000 biographies for the *Oxford Dictionary of National Biography*, 2004.
3 M. R. Currie (1997–98) 'Fever Nurses' Perceptions of their Fever Nurse Training 1921–1971', *International History of Nursing Journal*, 3(2): 5–19.
4 'Wills, probate', copy of John Fitzpatrick Villier's will, and other family wills obtained from Somerset House, London, 27 March 1997.
5 Archives and Museum, the Royal Hospitals NHS Trust, MO 54/2, Matron's report book on probationers, p.195.
6 KCLA/BCN2/10 Testimonial written by Isla Stewart, Matron and Superintendent of Nurses, St Bartholomew's Hospital, London, dated at the top, wrongly, 5 March 1897 (this date was changed in the middle of the reference to 1896).
7 Thompson (1990), p. 5.
8 Ayers (1971), p. 274.
9 Ibid., p. 18 (note 1) and p. 23.
10 McGann (1992), p. 60.
11 KCLA/RBNA/BCN2/11 Letter dated 6 May 1901, from Isla Stewart to Susan Villiers on her appointment as Matron of the Fountain Hospital.
12 NA/PRO DT10/173 Supplementary Register of Fever Nurses, no. 1. There are five such registers.
13 LMA, H9/GY/C4/2 Matron's Journal 1901–05, Guy's Hospital.
14 This concept arose again from time to time, particularly when the supplementary registers were being set up and after the inception of the NHS in 1948, when isolation hospitals began to close or change their use.
15 LMA MAB Minutes, 1909, XLIII, 163. A copy of the Syllabus of Lectures was published in *BJN*, 21 August 1909: 158.
16 Baly (1995), p. 152.
17 NA/PRO DT10/57 General Register of Nurses.
18 NA/PRO DT10/173 Supplementary Register of Fever Nurses, no. 1.
19 NA/PRO DT2/3 Part 2, Registrar's Reference File, GNC for England and Wales.
20 LMA MAB Minutes, 1924, vol. LVIII, p. 170.
21 Guild of St Barnabas Archive, *Misericordia*, June/July 1945, 64, 683, 3.

*———
Full references appear in the Bibliography.

22 LMA MAB 1165 Meeting of the Infectious Hospitals Committee; South Western Hospital Sub-Committee, June 1925 - December 1927, vol. 24.

23 *Kelly's Directory for Hertfordshire 1933*, p. 253.

24 NA/PRO C234/16 Crown Office: Fiats for Justices of the Peace, Hertfordshire, 1682–1929. Annie Villiers' name was inserted in the Commission of Peace for the County of Hertford, 9 March 1922. The Fiat was signed by Birkenhead C. I am indebted to Dr Ruth Paley, at the Public Record Office, now the National Archives, for this information. She stated that not all fiats survived, and that not everyone appointed sat then; it was just an honour to be a JP.

25 KCLA BCN/1 Minutes of the British College of Nurses, July 1926 - November 1927.

26 McGann (1992), p. 51.

27 Margaret Breay had also been a probationer and staff nurse at Bart's (1885–88), see KCLA/RBNA Books 3 General, *The Nursing Directory, or the Official Directory of Trained Nurses for 1909*. She would have been in training there when Miss Manson was Matron. This may be the reason for her being a life member as vice-president of the BCN appointed on 1 May 1926, the same day as Mrs Fenwick.

28 *Handbook of the National Council of Women of Great Britain (Federated to the International Council of Women in 1897), 1926–27*, p. 28. The Matrons' Council of Great Britain and Ireland was a body set up by Mrs Fenwick and Isla Stewart, intended to bring about a uniform system of nurse education in British hospitals. See McGann (1992), p. 42.

29 KCLA BCN 1/33 Minutes of the Meeting of 26 February 1927.

30 KCLA BCN 1/1 Minutes of the British College of Nurses, July 1926 – November 1927.

31 KCLA BCN 1/69 Twelfth Meeting of the Council, 25 June [1927].

32 KCLA, International Council of Nurses (ICN) 10/11 Brochure for Congress of the International Council of Nurses, Montreal, Canada, 8–13 July 1929, p. 1. No evidence has been found that she disputed this assertion.

33 KCLA, ICN 10/3/1 Letter to Margaret Breay from Susan Villiers, dated 30 July 1929.

34 KCLA, ICN 10/3/2 Letter to Margaret Breay from Susan Villiers, dated 6 August 1929.

35 Archives and Museum, the Royal Hospitals NHS Trust, SL6, *League News*, September 1942. Bart's was the first hospital to establish an association for trained nurses in Britain on the initiative of Isla Stewart, the Matron, who had been impressed by the alumnae associations in the United States. The first one there was founded in 1889 and by 1897 practically every training school in the United States had one. Bart's Nurses' League held its first meeting on 4 December 1899. 'The objectives were to encourage the members to strive for a high standard of work and conduct, the mutual help and pleasure of the members, and the establishment of a benevolent fund'. See McGann (1992), p. 67.

36 The Nurses Act, 1943, enabled the enrolment of assistant nurses, initially by experience, and subsequently, following a two-year course.

37 *BJN*, April 1945: 41.

38 In 2003, at the age of 79 years, she suffers from post-polio syndrome and has to wear calipers and a chest support. Jean is, apparently, a wonderful lady who has worked hard for polio victims all her life. She was a dressmaker and is also interested in history. She wrote a short booklet, *Belvoir Park Hospital: Fever 1840s–1986*, published privately in 1986.

39 Letter to the author, dated 16 June 2003.

40 Purdysburn Fever Hospital, 1904–48, changed its name twice: Northern Ireland Fever Hospital, 1948–75, and Belvoir Park Hospital, 1975–97.

41 Information from Harriet Cassells to author, 7 April 2004.

42 Mr Graham later became a nurse tutor after qualifying at the RCN in London, working first at the Northern Ireland Fever Hospital from 1967, until he took a post in 1975 as Senior Nurse Tutor at the North Down College of Nursing at Dundonald.

43 According to Kevin Brown (30 June 2003), the Archivist at St Mary's Hospital, Paddington and the author of the biography of Alexander Fleming (Brown, 2004), who discovered penicillin there in 1928, doctors and nurses in the Second World War commonly claimed that they saw or were the first to use penicillin. He feels it unlikely that a probationer nurse would be in a position to know this at the time - it could be hearsay or even interpretation after the event. However, there was a General Penicillin Committee for clinical use in selected cases that might advance knowledge of the properties of the drug. Certainly, the intramuscular route was a common means of administering penicillin in 1944–45.

44 Schedule for Harriet M. Thompson confirms date when training commenced - 19 October 1943; it also shows dates and areas in which she worked.

45 Copy of certificate awarded by Purdysburn Fever Hospital for the A. C. Cameron Prize, dated October 1946.

46 D. Guthrie (1945) *A History of Medicine*, London: Nelson.

47 Letter to author, dated 27 August 1995.

48 Baly (1980), p. 224.

49 Copies from RCNA and Harriet Cassells, FRCN, RFN, SRN.

50 *Nursing Standard*, 23 April 1985: 8.

51 *Belfast Telegraph*, 19 April 1985: 1.

52 Information sent to author, dated 2 May 2004.

53 Information sent to author, dated 10 May 2003.

54 Letter to author, dated 16 June 2003.

# 8  The aftermath of fever and smallpox nursing

It may seem a strange principle to enunciate as a first requirement in a hospital that it should do the sick no harm ... In all hospitals (and in a children's hospital much more than others) the patient must not stay a day longer than is absolutely necessary.

Florence Nightingale, *Notes on Hospitals*, 1863.[1]

## Introduction

The fever registers and the vast majority of isolation hospitals may have been closed in the United Kingdom and the Irish Republic by the early 1970s, but this left some nurses, particularly those with the single RFN qualification, in a quandary. The wisdom of establishing and maintaining isolation hospitals had been increasingly questioned in the twentieth century, but these institutions did not have a monopoly on infection, nor its control. The most feared of all infectious diseases, smallpox, was declared eradicated world-wide by the World Health Organisation in 1980, but the threat of bioterrorism means that it could re-emerge. In 1915, Mrs Bedford Fenwick used the phrase 'the aftermath of war' in relation to disabled soldiers. She wrote in terms of 'the onslaughts of a pitiless enemy'.[2] Metaphorical allusions to war, battles and struggles still permeate the literature in infectious disease control in the twenty-first century. It remains to be seen whether modern methods of infection control can defeat this 'pitiless enemy'. These issues are considered in the following sections to demonstrate that 'fevers' should not be underestimated. Nurses and others in the health care professions still need the necessary knowledge on which to base their practice, to prevent infection and cross-infection and provide safe care to enable patients to survive, whatever the circumstances.

## The single qualified nurse

It had never been the aim of the Fever Nurses' Association nor the GNC for England and Wales, that fever nursing should be a stand-alone qualification. Although some nurses assumed that they were able to work in any setting, it was a false premise which Susan Villiers, the new president of the FNA, strongly refuted in 1925. She stated then that such a nurse would remain 'a partially trained woman.'[3] When the GNCs assumed responsibility for training, fever nurse leaders lost their autonomy, but they banded themselves into professional associations, the League of Fever Nurses and the Infectious Hospitals Matrons' Association, from which they drew strength. They continued to struggle to achieve rights for the fever nurse, but following the closure of most isolation hospitals, they had little influence. Having failed to keep the Fever Register open, the reformed Infectious Hospitals Matrons' and Nurses' Association turned its attention to the status of the single qualified RFN, working in hospitals other than infectious diseases hospitals. A letter was sent on 5 April 1969 to the GNC for England and Wales, expressing concern about this matter. In her reply on 16 April, Miss M. Henry, Registrar, explained that these difficulties had concerned the GNC for some considerable time.

> In a situation which is no fault of the fever nurse, the conditions of employment laid down by the Whitley Council for their deployment and grading in fields other than fever nursing are quite unacceptable to the majority of fever nurses. Under the Whitley Council ruling a registered nurse employed in a field other than the one in which she is qualified, must be paid as an enrolled nurse . . . Nevertheless, the registered fever nurse cannot assume the status and qualification of an enrolled nurse . . . it is not possible for a registered fever nurse to become enrolled by virtue of her student nurse training in fever nursing since the Council would not grant two statutory qualifications in respect of one period of training. The only grade that remains available for this trained nurse is therefore that of an auxiliary.[4]

It is clear from Miss Henry's reply that the IHMNA had been concerned about the grading of a fever nurse as a nursing auxiliary, while being called upon to supervise and train pupil and student nurses. The GNC had, however, made representations to the Department of Health and Social Security in past years about the unsatisfactory position of the RFN, employed other than in that field of fever nursing. This could be overcome if they were granted the status and grading of a registered nurse with some salary adjustment, as had occurred with regard to a mental nurse employed in the field of mental subnormality. On 3 May 1969, the members of the IHMNA were informed of this unsatisfactory situation, which could seriously affect the career progression of the RFN, but no reply had been received from the Whitley Council.[5] However, on 22 September 1972, the Whitley Council issued a circular on the issue:

> a Senior Enrolled Nurse post may be filled where appropriate by a Registered Fever Nurse employed outside her speciality who is entitled

to be paid as an Enrolled Nurse ... provided that she has had the equivalent length and type of experience. Where she is filling such a post, the nurse concerned shall be paid as a Senior Enrolled Nurse.[6]

It is evident that widespread concern and efforts by various professional bodies had resulted in this gesture, which benefited some fever nurses, but as was seen in Chapter 4, other RFNs failed to secure a satisfactory conclusion.

## The wisdom of isolation hospitals

There had been debates about the wisdom of isolating patients in hospital for much of their existence. One issue concerned the spread of infection within isolation hospitals, referred to by an Edwardian cynic as a 'place where a person goes in with one infectious disease and catches all the rest'. Although Dr Caiger, an authoritative figure in the isolation hospital world, acknowledged in 1900 that the dreaded 'post-scarlatinal diphtheria' occurred more often in hospital than in home treatment, he still advocated mixing different infections in the same ward, provided that there was adequate ventilation, and sufficient floor space per bed. It is also known from Edwardian medical discussions of hospital reform that, in the past, poor practices contributed to hospital confinement, due to 'ignorance, carelessness and penury'. In some hospitals it was not unusual for one towel, one wash cloth or one tongue depressor to be used for an entire ward during the morning routine.[7]

It was clearly necessary for the education of fever nurses to develop to improve knowledge and understanding about cross-infection. In 1910, Miss Drakard, Matron of Plaistow Isolation Hospital, in the East End of London, noted that the first object of fever hospitals was to prevent the spread of various infections among the people, but also within them. She noted that 'patients suffering from different fevers may infect each other'.[8] However, it was the advances in bacteriology in the period 1890–1910 which had resulted in an emphasis on isolation and disinfection. In 1935, Dr W. G. Savage, the MOH for Somerset, deplored the vast sums spent on isolation hospitals; he believed that medical knowledge 'would render them unnecessary'.[9] This prophetic view was unlikely to have found favour with most MOHs, who as employees of local authorities, aided by legislation, had successfully argued for their establishment, overcoming councillors' concerns about costs; they, therefore, had a vested interest in their continued use.

The widespread belief that local MOHs preferred work related to curative rather than preventive medicine is exemplified in diphtheria prevention in Britain, which compared unfavourably with schemes in New York and some provinces in Canada. Immunisation with toxoid against diphtheria in the province of Ontario resulted in a fall in the death rate from 25.7 to 0.9 per 100,000 cases between 1920 and 1939. Although Britain was a world leader in improving diphtheria prophylaxis, it had one of the lowest immunisation rates. It was only in the Second World War that Ministry of Health officials, particularly concerned about the likelihood of epidemics in air-raid shelters, issued alum toxoid precipitate, first to the London boroughs, and a few weeks later, to all local authorities. This national campaign, backed up by films and posters, resulted in free immunisations, as local authorities were reimbursed by government funding, but the ministry insisted it was only 'a war service'. In 1943, the Chief Medical Officer noted that 50 per cent of the child population had been immunised in two years. The resultant decrease in the death rate was attributed entirely to the success of the national scheme.[10]

This important incursion into the nation's health, and the increasing use of antibiotics, sounded the death knell for isolation hospitals. As the Second World War drew to a close in 1945, a Sister Tutor at the LCC Park Fever Hospital reflected that 'this isolation system has not proved as effective in checking the spread of infection as was hoped'.[11] In 1953, the Medical Superintendent and the Matron of another large LCC fever hospital, Joyce Green Hospital, Dartford, Kent, noted the huge decline in infectious diseases:

> Patients are no longer incarcerated in fever hospitals for weeks to isolate them from the rest of the population. It is now known that isolation alone does not prevent, or materially alter, epidemics, so that hospital treatment is more concerned with the patient as an individual.[12]

Clearly, some individuals might still need specialist care when they contracted an infectious disease, but the consensus view was that containment of the masses in epidemics, particularly with childhood diseases, was no longer necessary. Dr W. M. Frazer, a Professor of Public Health at the University of Liverpool and MOH for the City and Port of Liverpool, wrote in 1950 that, communicable diseases, mainly by droplet infection, such as diphtheria, scarlet fever, measles, whooping cough and chickenpox were largely uncontrolled, even by the use of the isolation hospitals.[13] Following the rationalisation of hospital resources after 1948, patients could be sent to one of the regional units or transferred to special isolation units within general hospitals, where, because of reliance on the new antibiotics, it is possible that some routines, practised assiduously in fever hospitals, suffered, particularly hand-washing. In the period from the late 1960s, student nurses, like patients, were increasingly being seen as individuals. In an effort to retain them in general nurse training, the authoritarian approach, previously so familiar in fever and general hospitals, gradually began to give way to a more *laissez-faire* attitude. Strict obedience to hospital rules and regulations, with their punitive connotations, slowly gave way to less threatening 'procedures'. Moreover, it was difficult for hospitals, and matrons in particular, to retain their control of nurses when they moved away from nurses' homes to live in the community. The more relaxed attitude towards life in general and to authority did not augur well for the control of infection.

## Infection control nursing

The title 'fever nurse' may have been apt in the early nineteenth century, when infectious diseases were rife and their causation poorly understood, but it became increasingly outmoded by the mid-twentieth century. In fact, in the Irish Republic, a registered fever nurse was known as a registered infectious diseases nurse. As the need for, and belief in the wisdom of, isolation hospitals began to decline in the late 1940s, control of infection became more of an issue in general hospitals and other similar institutions. However, hospital acquired infections (HAIs) are not a new phenomenon. Before the use of disinfectants, antiseptics and aseptic wound dressing techniques, which developed following Joseph Lister's first use of carbolic acid in 1865,[14] there was widespread infection in general hospital wards. As wounds so commonly suppurated, the stench could permeate throughout the ward. Respectable, middle-class women were loath to nurse there and well-to-do patients preferred to be nursed at home, even if they required an operation. In 1863, Florence Nightingale wrote in *Notes on Hospitals*:

> Facts such as these [the high rate of infection and mortality in hospitals] have sometimes raised grave doubts as to the advantages to be derived from hospitals at all and have led many to think that in all probability a poor sufferer would have a much better chance of recovery if treated at home.[15]

It was the staphylococcus and streptococcus which commonly caused wound infections, often leading to gangrene. The haemolytic streptococcus was also responsible for some infectious diseases, including scarlet fever, erysipelas and puerperal (childbed) fever, much dreaded in maternity hospitals. Yet, although some wound infections and infectious diseases had the same causative organism, patients often had a different locus of care; those with the above-mentioned diseases were usually isolated in a fever hospital, while those with infections that they had acquired in a general hospital often remained there. In the Second World War hospital infections were still causing concern.

In 1944, the Medical Research Council (MRC) issued Memorandum 11, stating that every hospital should establish a Control of Cross Infection Committee, which 'should be the basis for standing orders which all hospital personnel would be required to know and obey'. In the late 1950s, some staphylococcal infections, particularly the virulent phage type 80, began to cause serious problems for patients and nurses. At that time, there was an increased incidence of staphylococcal infections in the nursing staff at the Torbay Hospital in Devon, which resulted in the appointment of the first infection control nurse (ICN). Other hospitals recognised the value of such a person and by the year 2000, there were over 600 ICNs in Britain, working in the public and private sectors and in military health care organisations. The first Infection Control Conference, held in 1966, became an annual event and the Infection Control Nurses' Association (ICNA) was established in 1970. Continuing education for these pioneering specialist nurses began in the late 1950s, by learning 'on the job' from the infection control doctor (ICD), who was usually a medical microbiologist. Gradually, courses of varying content, duration and complexity were developed and run by such professional bodies as the Joint Board of Clinical Nursing Studies and the English National Board. Since the transfer of all nurse education into higher education, which began in 1989, universities have validated their own courses at degree and master's level.[16] The University of Hertfordshire led the way in England, with Elizabeth Jenner, Principal Lecturer in Infection Control, devising, teaching and managing courses for specialist nurses. In 2002, the Royal College of Nursing honoured her with a fellowship for her work in infection control.[17]

ICNs have a broad remit, being not only part of an infection control team, but also expected to advise in clinical areas, carry out audits and teach student nurses and others. Unlike fever nurses, they are not constantly at the bedside. For this reason, existing staff have been appointed as link nurses in many hospital wards and departments, whose remit is to monitor standards, such as hand hygiene, and identify and report problems. The ICN's role as a specialist teacher involves considerable time in the preparation and delivery of lectures to students undergoing various nurse education programmes. As universities now validate their own basic nursing programmes, infection control input can vary.

In 2004, University of Luton students undergoing the adult/child branches had six hours in the common foundation programme (one year) on the introduction to infection control and hospital acquired infection. In the second year they had four hours on care of the immuno compromised patient, and surgery and the problems of infection, and in the third year they learned more about infection control from a management perspective, and intravenous therapy. There were also lectures from nurses in the Public Health Service (PHS), including the role of the PHS in promoting the health of communities and the population as a whole.[18]

Isolation hospitals and fever nurses no longer have the prerogative in caring for patients with infectious diseases, as infection exists in so many places and in so many forms. Wherever people gather together, especially in institutions, new viruses surface and old bacteria re-emerge, often in drug-resistant forms, like TB and Methicillin Resistant Staphylococcus Aureus (MRSA), which has now reached epidemic proportions to challenge nursing, medical and laboratory staff.

The bacterium staphylococcus aureus was first described in England in 1961, shortly after methicillin was introduced. Epidemic strains of the MRSA appeared in the 1990s. The incidence as a proportion of all S. Aureus blood cultures rose from under 5 per cent in 1991, to 42 per cent in 2000. Since 1990, the incidence of all S. Aureus bacteraemia due to MRSA in children has considerably increased; although not yet as high as in adults, it is becoming an increasing problem among children in England and Wales.[19]

MRSA is the commonest HAI. Its increased prevalence in adult and children's wards and departments is now creating public alarm in the same way as when earlier infectious diseases were spread within fever hospitals. The consumer magazine *Which?*, concerned about HAIs, particularly MRSA, carried out a survey by postal questionnaire in November 2003 of 5,000 acute care nurses in England, Wales, Scotland and Northern Ireland to ascertain how infections caught in hospitals are prevented and managed, and how hygiene practices are maintained. Only 806 nurses responded, a 16 per cent return rate, but, protected by confidentiality, some significant facts emerged. For instance, the study, published in the April 2004 edition of *Which?*, showed that seven in ten nurses blamed basic hygiene lapses in hospitals for many of the incidences of HAIs, including the so-called 'superbug' MRSA. A quarter of nurses in the study felt that insufficient toilet and bathing facilities contributed to HAIs in their hospitals.[20]

Control of infection is fundamental to care of the patient. It underlies modern criteria such as clinical governance and evidence-based practice, and as such plays a part in determining star ratings for NHS hospitals. Most hospitals now routinely swab patients transferred from other hospitals or elderly care homes. Should they prove positive to an infection, particularly MRSA, they can be isolated. Many hospitals segregate these patients in the side wards of a main ward, but a few, such as the Luton and Dunstable Hospital NHS Trust, have a designated isolation ward for MRSA patients. As elsewhere, there is an ongoing awareness about compliance with hand-washing policies, particularly for doctors and those carrying out nursing duties when moving between patients. Portable alcohol-based gels, carried by staff and in strategic positions, such as the notes' trolley and the ends of patients' beds, reduce the need to walk to distant basins for hand-washing. However, both methods still need to be carried out properly if they are to be effective in reducing cross-infection. Education, particularly by example, is the key.

In 2003, the government decided to play a part in trying to reduce the incidence of HAIs, particularly MRSA, through a raft of measures including boosting hygiene standards in hospitals. Those with the best and worst MRSA rates were named: they ranged from 0.04 cases per 1,000 'bed days' in the York Health Services Trust, compared to 0.30 cases in Weston Area Health. Directors of Infection Control now have the power to impose tough new rules on every hospital, and £3 million will be spent on research and development into HAIs.[21]

The control of infectious, or communicable, diseases is now a global issue. The medical and nursing press carry frequent articles on the subject and the media draw it to public attention. Hence, the WHO launched a World TB day on 24 March 2004, to revitalise political commitment and public participation in the global movement against tuberculosis. This disease now infects one-third of the world's population, but is curable in nearly all cases. Multidrug resistant TB remains low in the United Kingdom. The Human

Immunodeficiency Virus (HIV) continues to fuel the global TB problem, so the WHO has developed and expanded its strategy aimed at strengthening links between TB and HIV/AIDS (Acquired Immune Deficiency Syndrome). There is now evidence of a high prevalence of TB in prisons. TB nurses, health visitors, prison nurses and other specialist nurses are working together with medical and laboratory staff to identify problem areas, carry out surveillance studies and help patients.[22]

The media reported some of these issues in the national press. For example, the *Daily Mail* gave TB a whole page with an eye-catching headline, 'We're the TB capital', and a picture of children being checked for TB in 1938. This article includes most of the salient facts issued by the Health Protection Agency, such as TB cases have risen by almost 20 per cent in Britain between 1994 and 2003. In England and Wales there was a rise in cases from 5,798 in 1992 to 6,891 in 2002, with the Greater London boroughs among Britain's TB hot spots. Although levels have fallen in other western European nations, the infection is spreading in the United Kingdom as quickly as in eastern Europe. Lung physicians have repeatedly called for immigrants and long-stay visitors from countries rife with the disease to be screened on entry to Britain; they blame the increased incidence on a shortage of specialist doctors and nurses. Dr John Moore-Gillon, a TB specialist at the British Thoracic Society (BTS) called on the government to publish an action plan to focus on controlling infection rates.[23]

The *Daily Telegraph*, by contrast, gave 24 March little attention. The headline 'TB cases up 20 per cent in 10 years' headed three short paragraphs in the 'In Brief' column. It remarked that England and Wales were the only countries to see an increase, that the BTS attributed the rise to a combination of immigration and too few specialist doctors and nurses and showed the same statistics as the *Daily Mail*.[24]

Hospitals, with their infection control teams, struggle to cope, but in a different context from that in fever hospitals, where hospital rules and regulations were usually obeyed. The more relaxed, democratic approach in society today now hinders control of infection, despite infection control teams, link nurses and locally issued policies, based on centrally issued guidelines, which have to be followed. Those who fail to comply with hospital policies may be subject to disciplinary procedures. In the twenty-first century, the authoritarian approach is relatively rare, but non-compliance leaves the way wide open for infection, constantly lurking, waiting for an opportunity to develop.

As was seen earlier in Chapter 5, while the smallpox virus exists in laboratories, accidental infection could still occur. In August 2000, a postgraduate student, aged 24 years, researching a smallpox strain accidentally contracted a genetically modified variant of the highly infectious disease while carrying out a routine laboratory experiment at Imperial College London. Although he recovered, the late diagnosis in hospital, where he had been admitted to an open ward, could have put other patients and staff at risk. Doctor William

Carman, however, an expert in respiratory diseases at Glasgow University, stated that the likelihood of an outbreak was negligible as the viruses were not smallpox, but related to them and were designed not to spread from person to person.[25] It is important to remember that Great Britain, like other countries, now has a poorly protected population. Approximately half have never been vaccinated, as this practice stopped in the late 1970s, and even those who were would be susceptible because of their waning immunity. There is, therefore, the potential for a rapidly spreading epidemic which would require large-scale vaccination.[26]

In 2002 it became known that Russia still had the industrial facility capable of producing tons of smallpox virus annually. It also maintains a research programme that is believed to be trying to produce more virulent and contagious strains. An aerosol release of the smallpox virus would disseminate easily due to its considerable stability in aerosol form, and epidemiological evidence suggests the infectious dose is very small. As few as 50–100 cases of smallpox would probably result in widespread concern or panic and the need to implement large-scale or even national emergency measures. In 2000, the US Centers for Disease Control and Prevention awarded a contract for 40 million doses of smallpox vaccine.[27] In April 2002, the British Prime Minister, Tony Blair, hurried through an order for 16 million doses of smallpox vaccine after the US vice-president, Dick Cheney, warned him that a military attack on Iraq would result in a biological terror onslaught on Britain.[28] In October 2002, however, the Department of Health ruled out mass vaccination on the grounds that a nation-wide campaign could kill 60 people and harm many more. This viewpoint aroused considerable debate.[29]

The fear generated by potential bioterrorists attacks is, therefore, of international concern, demonstrated by the terrorist atrocity perpetrated on the World Trade Center in New York, on 11 September 2001, and the subsequent bioterrorist strikes with anthrax. The debate continues about the likelihood of an attack with smallpox virus, and also the risk involved in vaccination of large previously unprotected populations. Release of the virus would cause terror and the 'spreading epidemic could be fearsome'. As it spread world-wide, containment would be effective only in those countries with large supplies of vaccine and the medical infrastructure to deliver it.[30]

At a conference in Geneva on 21–22 October 2003, entitled 'Smallpox biosecurity: preventing the unthinkable', the delegates were left in no doubt that there will be new attempts to use biological agents in the twenty-first century. Apart from known stocks of the smallpox virus retained in laboratories in the United States and Russia, there is strong reason to believe that clandestine stocks are held in a number of other countries. Although the European Union has set up a rapid alert system for biological and chemical attack, only a few European countries have vaccine stockpiles and developing countries have made almost no preparations.[31] Although it may seem pessimistic to focus on potential epidemics, as the emergency services are aware, it is better to be prepared; lessons can be learned from the past.

## Conclusion

The importance of strong leadership in a smallpox epidemic was emphasised in Chapter 5, but it is unlikely that many nurses now would submit to the firm discipline imposed on them then, or be able, by virtue of their personal circumstances, to submit to quarantine. Segregation from society would be necessary, during the epidemic until the last patient had recovered, or after death if it occurred. Such social and professional isolation militates against harmony in the home and career development. Not only is it a more secular society today, where vocation is scarcely mentioned, but also it is a more litigious one. Occupational diseases affecting nurses, such as 'bad backs' and 'allergies', now carry with them the threat of litigation and compensation. No evidence has been found of such factors in the cases of those who sacrificed their health or lives in the nineteenth and twentieth centuries to infectious diseases, particularly smallpox.

Future national and local policies concerning serious communicable diseases should be formulated by a multidisciplinary team, including academics and clinical nurse specialists in control of infection. There can be no excuse for accepting nurses who volunteer to work in hazardous epidemic situations who are not fully protected by vaccination, cognisant of all the features of the disease and aware of the consequences. Their consent in writing should be given only when safe working practices have been agreed. There is still no proven antiviral agent effective in the treatment of smallpox. Supportive therapy and antibiotics for secondary bacterial infections are all that are available. Nursing care, for different forms of infectious disease, remains an essential service to individuals and for the health, prosperity and well-being of the nation.

## Notes and references*

1 Baly (1997), pp. 58–59.
2 *BJN*, 30 January 1915: 81.
3 *BJN,* June 1925: 124.
4 RCNA C337/3 Letter dated 16 April 1969, to Miss R. M. Rogers, Honorary Secretary, IHMNA, from Miss M. Henry, Registrar, GNC for England and Wales. The letter sent by the IHMNA is not in this archive.
5 RCNA C337/5 IHMNA Minutes of the Executive Meeting, 3 May 1969, at the Infectious Diseases Hospital, Devonshire Road, Blackpool.
6 RCNA C337/3 NMC Circular no. 165, Whitley Councils for the Health Services (Great Britain), Nurses and Midwives Council. Definition of Senior Enrolled Nurse, 22 September 1972.
7 J. M. Eyler (1987) 'Scarlet Fever and Confinement: the Edwardian Debate over Isolation Hospitals', *Bulletin of the History of Medicine*, 61: 1–24.

*———

Full references appear in the Bibliography.

8 M. Drakard (1910) 'The Nurse in Fever Hospitals', *Nursing Times*, 5 November: 906.

9 Lewis (1986), pp. 5, 28.

10 J. Lewis (1986) 'The Prevention of Diphtheria in Canada and Britain 1914–1945', *Journal of Social History*, 20: 163–76.

11 Watson (1945), p. 2.

12 M. Mitman and E. M. Couzins (1953) 'Fever Training in a General Hospital', *Nursing Mirror*, 13 March: xi.

13 Frazer (1950), p. 364.

14 Porter (1997), p. 371.

15 Baly (1997), p. 61.

16 E. A. Jenner and J. A. Wilson (2000) 'Educating the Infection Control Team - Past, Present and Future. A British Perspective', *Journal of Hospital Infection*, 46: 96–105.

17 Interview with Ms Jenner at the University of Hertfordshire, 25 November 2003.

18 Schedule of Lectures, 'Infection Control Input to Project 2000 Programme - University of Luton' from Sue Fox, Senior Infection Control Nurse, Luton and Dunstable Hospital NHS Trust, Luton, dated 12 February 2003, and the University of Luton Student Handbook, September 2003, Diploma in Higher Education (Nursing): Registered Nurse.

19 N. Khairulddin, L. Bishop, T. L. Lamagni, M. Sharland and G. Duckworth (2004) 'Emergence of Methicillin Resistant Staphylococcus Aureus (MRSA) Bacteraemia among Children in England and Wales, 1990–2001', *Archives of Disease in Childhood*, 89(4): 378–79.

20 *Which?*, 'The Curse of the Superbug', April 2004: 10–13, and Royal College of Nursing (2004) 'The Fight against Hospital Infections', *rcnbulletin*, 7–20 April.

21 Press release: reference 2003/0500, Department of Health, and *BBC NEWS* | Health ' "Superbug" Crackdown is Launched', 9 December 2003: 1–4.

22 HPA Tuberculosis Update 2004, http://www.hpa.org.uk/infections/topics_az/tb/menu.htm

23 *Daily Mail*, 24 March 2004.

24 *Daily Telegraph*, 24 March 2004.

25 *Daily Mail*, 18 December 2000: p. 18.

26 D. A. Henderson (2000) 'Smallpox Virus Destruction', *Biodefense News*, http://www.hopkins-biodefense.org/pages/news/research.htm/(18 April 2000).

27 'Smallpox' Fact Sheet Info. Center for Civilian Biodefense Strategies, http://www.hopkins-biodefense.org/pages/agentsmallpox.html/(23 January 2003).

28 *Sunday Telegraph*, 14 April 2002: 4. This catastrophe did not occur.

29 *Daily Telegraph*, 10 October 2002: 16.

30 R. T. Johnson (2003) 'Smallpox: The Threat of Bioterrorism and the Risk of the Vaccine', *Neurology*, 60: 1228–29.

31 'Conference Highlights Bioterrorist Threat', *Lancet*, 362, 25 October 2003: 1386.

# 9   Conclusion

There is much more work to be done in the history of nursing.
Celia Davies (1980)[1]

This aphorism sums up this particular nursing history. More could have been included from research already carried out and, almost certainly, more will be revealed by others as additional evidence comes to light. History is not finite. Fever (isolation) hospitals were established in nineteenth-century Britain to meet a particular need – control of epidemics, by the removal and isolation of people with infectious diseases from the general population, but the new system was also part of a movement to medicalise care. However, reservations began to be expressed about the wisdom of their existence in the twentieth century, and public opinion began to change until it was thought they were no longer necessary. The service was maintained only because fever nurse probationers made such a valuable contribution to the health of the British nation by staffing the hospitals and, through training, gradually gave the patient better and more specialised care, truly a service to the nation.

The transition from community to institutional care was a slow process, and the infinite variety in the size of fever hospitals and the nursing practices which prevailed, impacted on standards of nursing care. Faced initially in the early to mid-nineteenth century, 'the dark era of nursing', with poorly educated, immoral and untrained women, they were transformed by compulsory elementary education, better conditions of service, improved pay and nurse training, into professional nurses, a situation very similar to that in general nursing. There was no national scheme to establish fever hospitals in the nineteenth century, but nevertheless, they were set up, where they were most needed, in and around large urban areas and ports. The Metropolitan Asylums Board in London provided a nearly perfect model of institutional provision from the 1870s, to control epidemics of common infectious diseases and smallpox, and it managed to stamp out the variola major form of small-pox by c.1901–02.

The Isolation Hospitals Acts, 1893, 1901, and the Notification Acts, 1889, 1899, and other legislation resulted in the, often reluctant, establishment of institutions by far smaller local authorities in England and Wales. The situation was different, in some respects, in Scotland and Ireland, partly because the population was smaller and more widely scattered, although large cities such as Glasgow, Edinburgh and Dublin met the need for fever hospitals at an early date. However, in the nineteenth century, and in some cases beyond, many patients in Britain with infectious diseases were accommodated in workhouses, or poorhouses, most of which later had infirmaries. Wherever they were to be found, due to the associations of poverty, and fear of the disease, fever patients were stigmatised, and in some areas, pauperised. It is clear that fever hospitals could not have coped in epidemics without Poor Law infirmaries, which frequently took excess patients.

Many small authorities had railed against burdening ratepayers with the expense of establishing and maintaining hospitals which were often underoccupied or empty, but in epidemics were often inadequate. However, once convinced that they were an asset, they became proud of their municipal munificence and were more likely to agree to new developments, such as cubicles, instead of open wards. However, concern had been expressed concerning cross-infection in isolation hospitals (although cubicalisation was a useful preventive strategy). Care at home was increasingly seen as a viable alternative, except for the seriously ill.

During the period up to, and in some cases after the Second World War, social class and status were paramount in isolation hospitals. It manifested itself in the type of residential accommodation allocated, uniform worn by the nurses and the tasks they were given. Probationers were the backbone of the service. Without their labour it could not have survived. However, they could not have functioned without nurse leaders, both in management and education and similarly, it appears, they needed support and advice. Medical men have been seen to be most supportive; it was clearly in their best interests to have a trained workforce to carry out their orders.

Certain doctors were particularly helpful in establishing professional fever nursing in the early twentieth century, including in London, Dr Biernacki, of the Plaistow Isolation Hospital, the founder of the FNA in 1908, Dr Goodall and Dr Caiger from MAB hospitals, and in Manchester, Dr Knyvett Gordon, from the University of Manchester. Of course, without the goodwill and financial support of her husband, Dr Bedford Fenwick, it is unlikely that Mrs Fenwick would have had the resources to edit and contribute to her own journal, the *British Journal of Nursing*, and campaign for state registration, in which fever nurse leaders became involved. Mrs Fenwick's importance in the professionalisation of nursing, including fever nursing, is apparent in this text.

The role of nursing journals should not be underestimated. They provided contemporary nurses with useful information on matters of professional interest and present-day historians with valuable evidence. The consensus view of most medical men and the majority of fever nurse leaders was that all nurses should be trained in fevers as epidemics were still common in the early twentieth century. However, the sheer volume of nurses and patients, spread across so many institutions, prevented this being put into practice. The best solution was found to be a fever course first, then general training, but this was not possible for everyone.

Medical men came from a higher social sphere, as did some early nurse leaders mentioned here, including Mrs Fenwick, Eva Lückes, Isla Stewart, Susan Villiers and Edith Cavell. By the twentieth century, the role of matron in many large hospitals had been transformed from that of housekeeper to inspector of standards and controller of nurses and nurse training. In small hospitals, the roles were more blurred; matrons lent a hand anywhere. Nevertheless, they and doctors expected, and received, deference and obedience from the lower orders. As doctors usually had the greater knowledge, they gave lectures, wrote textbooks and guided their fever nurse colleagues towards regulation of their profession in 1919, which they had already achieved through the Medical Act, 1858. As the twentieth century progressed, fever nurse matrons and tutors became more confident, independent and knowledgeable, they gave lectures, and they wrote textbooks. In epidemics, where careful conscientious nursing was more important than medical intervention, strong capable women emerged to take control. Examples have been given, particularly in smallpox outbreaks, and in the late nineteenth century, a woman who transformed nursing care in a fever hospital in Glasgow, without the benefit of nurse training, because she was a good organiser.

Fever hospitals existed in the United States, but fever nursing did not develop as a specialism there with separate nurse education and registration, unlike the British model of a separate branch of nursing, which evolved slowly over the nineteenth century. Most British entrants then had only an elementary education. Once courses began, better educated women were admitted for training and probationers were able to apply theory to practice. By the time fever nurses were qualified, they were experts, or specialists, in their field and, as the twentieth century progressed, some, like Harriet Cassells, were used in a consultative role to other hospitals. 'Paying probationers', well-educated women of a higher social class who paid for the privilege of a few months' nursing experience in general nursing, did not appear to exist in fever nursing. All social classes entered as equals, undertook the same training and were subjected to the same risks to their health. Until the early twentieth century, isolation hospitals were mostly used by the poor, but as confidence in them grew, more middle-class and well-to-do patients were admitted; it was rare for upper-class or really wealthy patients to opt for hospital care as provision could be made at home. However, the London Fever Hospital served the needs of some as it was a voluntary hospital and regarded differently from the municipal hospitals used mainly by 'the lower orders'.

It is not wise to generalise about why people wanted to work in isolation hospitals, but there is some evidence that better educated girls, such as those with a grammar school education, went to large hospitals, some of which had preliminary training schools, and those who left school earlier, to small hospitals, where nurses went straight on to wards and learned in apprentice fashion. Better pay and conditions made the difference, but few girls had careers' advice; often particular hospitals were recommended by word of mouth. Although they wanted a training, like the men who applied after the Second World War, they also needed to earn their living; fever nurse probationers were employees, not truly students. Men came into fever nursing too late to make any appreciable difference, as they had in pay and conditions in mental nursing; it is not known to what extent patients benefited, but male RFNs almost certainly gained from the experience professionally.

Fever nurses may have achieved state registration in 1919, but it was on one of the less prestigious supplementary registers. Parallels may be seen during the Second World War, when experienced assistant nurses, who bore the brunt of the work in general hospitals and public assistance infirmaries, were also given state recognition, not on the register, but on a roll, through the Nurses Act, 1943. Both involved two-year courses and, it seems, both suffered, at times, from superior attitudes from those who had undertaken a three year course. The single qualified RFNs received only limited help from the GNC for England and Wales when isolation hospitals closed. Some had difficulty in finding work and became disillusioned with nursing. Recruitment and retention of probationers was difficult, particularly in small hospitals not approved for training, where registration was not possible.

A number of examples have been given of nurses contracting and, sometimes, succumbing to the same infectious diseases as their patients, despite prophylactic measures. It is not clear if women as young as 16–17 years old, the age at which they were taken on from the 1930s, were truly aware of the risks they were taking. The extra leave awarded after some epidemics, particularly of smallpox, and the higher rate of pay fever nurses commanded in some large hospitals may have been personal compensation, but it was actually an acknowledgment that fever and smallpox hospitals were hazardous places in which to work.

Occupationally acquired conditions were different from those which concern nurses and management today. 'Bad backs' and stress-related problems did not figure large in isolation hospitals. By the 1930s, most of the heavy work was carried out by strong young women; there were rarely problems with finances or their personal lives as they all lived in, in a sheltered, but somewhat cloistered, environment. Consequently, time and money were not spent travelling to work; until after the Second World War fever nurses seldom tried to juggle a training course with marriage and children. As was seen, fever nurses were mostly expected to obey orders and work within the boundaries of hospital rules and regulations, although it is by no means certain that all hospitals had them. However, when medical men were not there, or when on ambulance duty, nurses were expected to manage in emergencies. Evidence has shown that sufficient expertise and management skills developed during the second year of training to cope with most eventualities.

Some very good examples of fever nurses' lifestyle and their attitudes, which prevailed in the period 1921–71, were given in Chapter 4. Their descriptions of nursing care are of great value in the history of this specialism. It is clear that many were self-sacrificing; they often put their personal social lives on hold, sublimating their own needs during training, but were compensated by the camaraderie, which often led to lifelong friendships. Heroism has been mentioned at times, but they did not use the term themselves. Those who could stand the long hours and hard work, often under a strict authoritarian régime, remained to complete their course. Most seemed compassionate and devoted to duty and saw the care of very ill patients as their vocation; their patients' recovery, if it happened, was their reward. Living-in had advantages for nurses, who could always find someone with a listening ear, and for managers, as nurses were instantly available in epidemics and there was less need to employ costly agency nurses. The needs of the service were paramount, hence when probationers were needed in other wards, they were moved, thus disrupting their planned experience: they were 'pairs of hands'.

The rarely heard patient impact narratives give added weight to Goffman's concerns about institutionalisation. Certainly, from the patient's perspective it is possible to see analogies between incarceration in asylums and prisons, and in some isolation hospitals, where they were mostly deprived of visitors, a factor particularly disturbing to children, who formed the main part of the patient population. In this study, individuals have been seen to make a difference, whether rank and file nurses, like those in the 1921–71 research study, or people like Susan Villiers, in management, Harriett Cassells in the clinical situation and, more recently, Elizabeth Jenner in education. Each in their own way contributed to patients' recovery and thus lowered mortality rates; moreover, they furthered the profession of nursing.

It became clear as the research continued and findings emerged, that there were considerable variations in the standards of care possible in large and small hospitals because of the resources they could command. Large hospitals had better qualified medical staff, resident on site, and nurses who had specialised as a result of approved courses and were better equipped to teach probationers, some of whom had the benefit of preliminary training. Technical innovations were carried out when first discovered and up-to-date equipment and accommodation for staff was provided.

As was seen, small hospitals were unlikely to gain approval for training; their nurses were disadvantaged and it is likely that patient care suffered at times. These factors may have contributed to the lack of trust in small rural hospitals, where the public took longer to gain confidence. It seems that stigma, associated with fear, and deaths of people in hospital known to all in the locality, were major contributory factors. Ignorance also played a large part in their delayed acceptance. Unlike the general public in Germany, many people in Britain ignored the need for vaccination against smallpox and immunisation against diphtheria yet, when they became seriously ill, wanted hospital admission. Because of this factor, a fatalistic attitude towards illness, and because early signs and symptoms were not recognised, the patient could be concealed at home and the doctor called in too late for any measures taken by the hospital to be effective. These were mostly young lives, valued not just by their families, but by the nation.

The permissive nature of some legislation, such as the Isolation Hospitals Act, 1893, meant that local areas could decide whether to set up training schemes in any small hospitals they founded, but no guidelines were issued by central government. Large hospitals had to think on a grander scale, but even the MAB failed to approve the FNA nurse training scheme in its hospitals until 1909. As was seen, Scotland and Ireland both set up their own national fever nurse training schemes before state registration finally became a reality. These early initiatives, particularly in Scotland, which decided on a three-year fever nurse course, unlike England and Wales and Ireland, delayed standardisation and caused professional rifts.

The irony of fever nursing is, that having struggled to establish and improve patient care, fever nurses were no longer needed; the Second World War provided the necessary impetus for change. Properly organised immunisation campaigns against diphtheria, and the gradual introduction of penicillin, transformed the care of patients with streptococcal infections. The decreased usage of hospital wards showed that, apart from diseases like poliomyelitis and laryngeal diphtheria in unimmunised children, isolation hospitals had mainly outlived their usefulness. However, as was seen in Chapter 7, Harriet Cassells in Belfast was just beginning her fever nursing career then; she, and her contemporaries, provided a service caring for patients in Northern Ireland for many years after the war.[2] The locus of care for patients with infectious diseases and their nurses changed when the hospitals closed. However, from the patients' and nurses' perspectives, a wider range of up-to-date resources and services became available. Redundant fever hospitals, freed of their patients, could serve their community in some other capacity, perhaps for convalescent or frail, elderly patients, or meet some other local need. Nurses, now divorced from their known setting, may have found it hard to adjust, but there was often access to continuing education and more opportunity to socialise. Change, therefore, ultimately benefited everyone, except, perhaps for some single qualified fever nurses.

Fever nurses saved lives. It was their misfortune that scientific advances, antitoxins, vaccines and antibiotics, plus better living standards and nutrition, resulted in closure of isolation hospitals and fever registers and ended their specialist practice. However, their knowledge and expertise were welcomed in general hospitals, where some nurses found employment in infection control. Cross-infection with hospital acquired infections, the burgeoning problem in general hospitals today, provided new challenges. If there are any lessons to be learned, it is that specialisation can be fraught with problems when the needs of society change. Nursing has to adapt as much now as it ever did, according to the expectations of society and the needs of patients, wherever they are found.

This study has shown that insufficient data were collected and collated centrally to enable standards of care to be monitored. For example, no national statistics were kept on the effectiveness of care in hospital versus the patient's own home in the form of morbidity/mortality figures, and there was a similar paucity concerning fever nurses who had contracted infectious diseases. This lack of quantative data hampered some conclusions being drawn. However, some new evidence has come to light, particularly nursing care knowledge directly from the nurses involved. As most patients were in hospital for many weeks, fever nurses got to know them well and were able to enhance their powers of observation, a faculty deemed most desirable by Florence Nightingale. Due to long hours of duty at the bedside, their special senses were well developed; they identified diseases by their rashes, could predict the outcome of some fevers by temperature and by listening to changed respirations and could recognise some diseases, particularly diphtheria, by the smell of the patient's breath.

Access to primary sources, together with considerable evidence from some of the 127 respondents in the 1921–71 case study, led to the conclusion that many fever nurses in twentieth-century Britain were ruled with a rod of iron. Some matrons and ward sisters had served in the First or Second World Wars, hence their military manner. Strict obedience to rules and regulations may now seem unnecessarily officious, but it was done with a purpose, usually to prevent cross-infection between patients and between patients and nurses. Relatives were also strictly controlled, with bedside visiting mostly forbidden. Talking to patients, and seldom giving them explanations about their care and progress, was also frowned upon in some hospitals. Bed-bathing patients from 2 a.m. must surely have seemed inappropriate, but nurses mostly did as they were bid. Obedience may be fine, but unquestioning compliance to doctors' orders can, in some circumstances, be dangerous. An extreme example in Germany led to nurses' involvement and complicity in the annihilation of patients declared to be unworthy by the state in the Third Reich (1933–45). As Hilde Steppe, who carried out extensive research in this period, wrote, 'nursing has the right and also the duty to treat humanely all who require nursing assistance'.[3] In Britain, the physical needs of fever patients took priority over psychological needs. Psychology was late to enter the curriculum.

Strict discipline and proper attention to personal hygiene, particularly hand-washing, were emphasised: they helped prevent cross-infection among patients and minimised the risk to fever nurses. A major finding in this study was the emphasis placed on obedience, essential when fever nurses were uneducated; rules and regulations were followed. As the twentieth century progressed and fever hospitals closed, the more relaxed attitudes in society pervaded general hospitals. Despite better educated doctors and nurses, a reluctance to respond to authoritarian régimes was apparent; one reason, perhaps, for HAIs becoming more difficult to control. Many patients are now better educated, aware of their rights and reluctant to accept poor hygiene standards meekly.

Society, however, has not changed much over the centuries in its attitudes to infectious diseases and, to a certain extent, those who provide care for those affected. Lepers and those with the plague and smallpox were cast outside the confines of the community. The once feared old-style vagrants, because of their tendency to spread smallpox, may have virtually disappeared, but others now threaten the health of the British nation.

In the twenty-first century, itinerants are very visible in urban streets: the asylum-seekers, homeless and dropouts from society. These people are now causing concern due to the rise in the incidence of HIV/AIDS and drug-resistant strains of tuberculosis. Although this book has touched on some aspects of nursing care of those with venereal diseases, now termed sexually transmitted diseases, including some mention of lock hospitals, they really demand their own in-depth study. Tuberculosis has been the focus of a number of medico-historical narratives and theses, but no work exists from a nursing/patient perspective. This study has shown, as Celia Davies prophesied in 1980, that 'There is much more work to be done in the history of nursing'; certainly considerable data exist for both these conditions. It has been possible only to touch on potential threats of bioterrorism from a global perspective, but this issue also needs addressing from a nursing, not just a political perspective.

Since 1860, nursing gradually became a respected profession in Britain. It evolved differently from the United States and other countries, but there can be little doubt that fever nursing served the needs of society. Fever nursing was the only branch of nursing in Britain which was founded for a specific reason, in the nineteenth century, carried out its objective and had a definite conclusion. Fever hospitals and fever nurses served their original purpose, the preservation of life for people who were not infected, in fact, a national service.

## Notes and references*

1  Davies (1980), p. 17.
2  Belvoir Park Hospital from 1975.
3  H. Steppe (1997) 'Nursing under Totalitarian Regimes: the Case of National Socialism', in Rafferty et al. (1997), pp. 10-27.

*————

Full references appear in the Bibliography.

# Appendix 1 Notifiable diseases in England and Wales (with the date each was made notifiable under current or similar nomenclature)

|  | *When made notifiable* |
|---|---|
| **Under the Public Health (Control of Disease) Act, 1984** | |
| Cholera | 1889 |
| Food poisoning | 1949 |
| Plague | 1900 |
| Relapsing fever | 1889 |
| Smallpox | 1889 |
| Typhus | 1889 |
| **Under the Public Health (Infectious Diseases) Regulations, 1988** | |
| Acute encephalitis | 1918 |
| Acute poliomyelitis | 1912 |
| Anthrax | 1960 |
| Diphtheria | 1889 |
| Dysentery (amoebic or bacillary) | 1919 |
| Leprosy | 1951 |
| Leptospirosis | 1968 |
| Malaria | 1919 |
| Measles | 1940 |
| Meningitis | 1968 |
| Meningococcal septicaemia (without meningitis) | 1988 |
| Mumps | 1988 |
| Ophthalmia neonatorum | 1914 |
| Paratyphoid fever | 1889 |
| Rabies | 1976 |
| Rubella | 1988 |
| Scarlet fever | 1889 |
| Tetanus | 1968 |
| Tuberculosis | 1912 |
| Typhoid fever | 1889 |
| Viral haemorrhagic fever | 1976 |
| Viral hepatitis | 1968 |
| Whooping cough | 1940 |
| Yellow fever | 1968 |

Source: A. McCormick (1993) 'The Notification of Infectious Diseases in England and Wales', *Communicable Disease Review*, 3(2), R20.

# Appendix 2 The first Governing Body of the Fever Nurses' Association, 1908

| | |
|---|---|
| President: | Dr Goodall, Medical Superintendent, Eastern Hospital, MAB |
| Vice-presidents: | Dr Pearson, Medical Superintendent, City Hospitals, Leeds |
| | Dr Brownlee, Physician-Superintendent, Belvidere Hospital, Glasgow |
| | Mrs Doran, Matron, City Hospitals, Leeds |
| | Miss Drakard, Matron, Plaistow Hospital |
| Hon. Treasurer: | Dr Caiger, Medical Superintendent, South Western Hospital, MAB |
| Hon. Secretaries: | Dr Biernacki, Medical Superintendent, Plaistow Hospital |
| | Miss Morgan, Matron, Northern Hospital, MAB |
| Members of Council: | *Medical Superintendents* |
| | Dr Broad, Cardiff Sanatorium |
| | Dr Mullen, Ladywell Sanatorium, Salford |
| | Dr Maccombie, Brook Hospital, MAB |
| | Dr Love, Fever Hospital, Greenock |
| | Dr Rhodes, Baguley Sanatorium, Manchester |
| | Dr Rundle, City Hospital, Fazakerley, Liverpool |
| | Dr Stewart, Fever Hospital, Willesden |
| | Dr Turner, South Eastern Hospital, MAB |
| | Dr Williams, City Hospital, Sheffield |
| | *Medical Officers of Health* |
| | Dr McCleary, Hampstead |
| | Dr Butler, Willesden |
| | Dr Corbin, Stockport |
| | Dr Clark, Assistant MOH, Leeds |
| | *Hospital Medical Officers of Health* |
| | Dr Cameron, South Eastern Hospital, MAB |
| | Dr Ta 'Bois, South Western Hospital, MAB |

*Matrons*
Miss Clarke, City Hospital, Fazakerley, Liverpool
Miss Gregory, London Fever Hospital
Miss Hay, Cardiff Sanatorium
Miss Ambler-Jones, South Eastern Hospital, MAB
Miss M. Jones, Gore Farm Hospital, MAB
Miss M. Lloyd, North Western Hospital, MAB
Miss Carson Rae, Cork Street Fever Hospital, Dublin
Miss A. Thomas, Park Hospital, MAB
Miss K. Thomas, Ladywell Sanatorium, Salford
Miss Villiers, Fountain Hospital, MAB
Miss Watkinson, Fever Hospital, Norwich
Miss Aitken, Belvidere Hospital, Glasgow
Miss Bond, Fever Hospital, Croydon
Miss Stevenson, Fever Hospital, Huddersfield
*Assistant Matrons*
Miss Bryson, Northern Hospital, MAB
Miss Winmill, South Western Hospital, MAB

Source: *British Journal of Nursing*, 11 July 1908: 30.
Note: Of the thirty-nine geographically well-spread representatives, twenty were doctors, nineteen were nurses. The Metropolitan Asylums Board in London was represented by six doctors and eight nurses, 36 per cent of the total number.

# Appendix 3  Advertisements for probationers for fever hospitals in England and Wales, 1919

| Name of hospital | Number registered | Minimum age | Other requirements | Salary per annum | Uniform | Applications to: | Benefits |
|---|---|---|---|---|---|---|---|
| Isolation Hospital, Brechin, N B (30 beds) | One at once | 18–20 years | | £20 and £25 | Part uniform | The Matron | |
| Kingsthorpe Isolation Hospital, Northampton (32 beds) | Two | Not under 20 years | | £24 rising by £3 yearly to £36 | £5 provided per annum | MOH, Guildhall, Northampton | |
| Walthamstow Urban Isolation Hospital, Chingford Hatch, E4 (84 beds) | | | Healthy and well educated | £22 1st year £24 2nd year | Provided | The Matron, with photo and recent references | Lectures. Certificate of the FNA after examination. War bonus £13 p.a. |
| Isolation Hospital, East Ham, E6 (98 beds) | | | Strong, well educated | £20 1st year £23 2nd year £26 3rd year | Indoor uniform provided | The Matron, with three recent testimonials and photograph | Three years training certificate. (Lectures) War bonus £15 |
| Sanatorium, Huddersfield (120 beds) | | 20 years | | £23 £25 inc. bonus | Materials for uniform | The Matron | Two years fever and tuberculosis training |
| Monsall Fever Hospital, Manchester (365 beds) | | 19 years | Well educated, of sound health | £20 1st year £25 2nd year | Indoor uniform | The Matron | Two years training. Lectures and certificate. |
| MAB Fever Hospitals, London<br>– Eastern, Homerton, E9 (375 beds)<br>– North Western, Hampstead, NW3 (464 beds)<br>– Park Hospital, Lewisham, SE13 (548 beds)<br>– North Eastern, South Tottenham, N15 (623 beds) | | 19 years | Good education | £40 1st year £42 2nd year | | The Matron | Fever certificate after passing necessary examination. Facilities to enter General Hospitals to complete training for those who do well. |

Sources: *Nursing Mirror and Midwives' Journal*, 30 August 1919 and *Burdett's Hospitals and Charities*, 1919.

# Appendix 4 Certificates

No. *1929*.

FEVER NURSES' ASSOCIATION.

Certificate of Registration.

THIS IS TO CERTIFY that

Mrs. *Fanny Elizabeth Ody.*

has passed the necessary examination and is duly registered
by the Fever Nurses' Association as a trained Fever Nurse.

*John Beswick* M.D. DSc.,
President.

*Egerton H. Williams.* M.D.
Acting Chairman of Education Committee.

*A. C. Tabois.*

*L. A. Morgan.*
Joint Hon. Secretaries.

Date *April 6. 1915*

SEAL OF THE ASSOCIATION.

NOTE.—This Certificate of Registration remains valid only so long as the permanent
address of the holder is known to the honorary secretaries. Any change of address should
therefore be notified to one of the honorary secretaries without delay.

4.1 Fever Nurses' Association Certificate of Registration, 1915: Fanny
Elizabeth Ody.

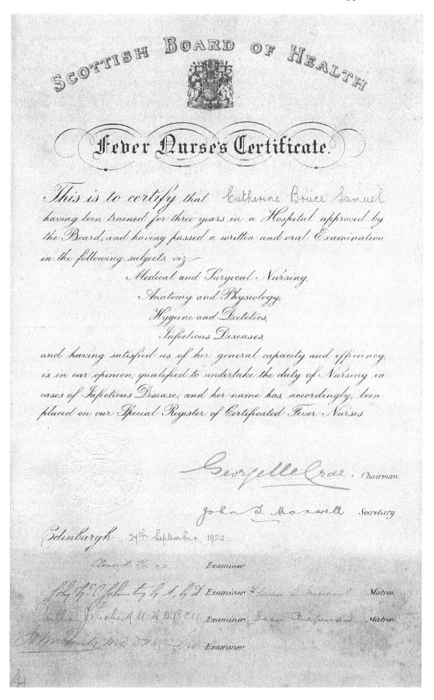

4.2 Scottish Board of Health Fever Nurse's Certificate, 1920: Catherine Bruce Samuel.

4.3 Metropolitan Asylums Board Certificate of Fever Training, North Western Fever Hospital, 1922: Ethel Mayo Hancock.

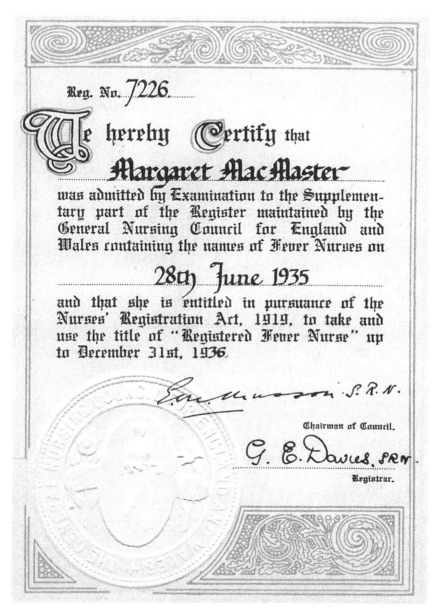

Reg. No. 7226

Ꮤe hereby Certify that

**Margaret MacMaster**

was admitted by Examination to the Supplementary part of the Register maintained by the General Nursing Council for England and Wales containing the names of Fever Nurses on

**28th June 1935**

and that she is entitled in pursuance of the Nurses' Registration Act, 1919, to take and use the title of "Registered Fever Nurse" up to December 31st, 1936.

*S.R.N.*

Chairman of Council.

*G. E. Davies, SRN.*

Registrar.

4.4 General Nursing Council for England and Wales, 1935: Margaret MacMaster.

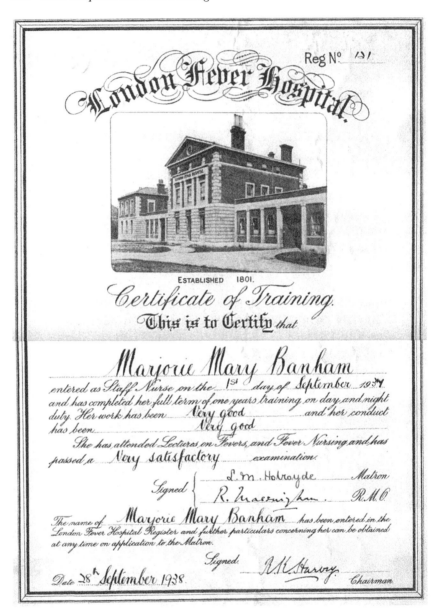

4.5 London Fever Hospital Certificate of Training, 1938: Marjorie Mary Banham.

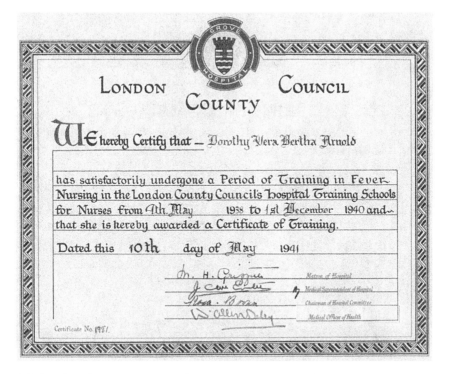

4.6 London County Council, Grove Hospital, 1941: Dorothy Vera Bertha Arnold.

No. *12*

## Dunstable & District Hospital Joint Committee

·········································

**This is to Certify** that *Olive Cowley*

entered the Committee's Hospital as a Probationer on the *First* day of

*February*, 1942, and left on the *First* day

of *February*, 1944, and that during that time she conducted

herself and performed her duties satisfactorily.

Dated the *19*th day of *January* 1944.

*Charles J. Kilby* ___Chairman

*J. B. Kume,* ___Medical Officer

*Gertrude Dobson.* ___Matron

*Countersigned by*

*J. B. Road* ___Clerk to the Committee

4.7 Dunstable and District Hospital Joint Committee, 1944: Olive Cowley.

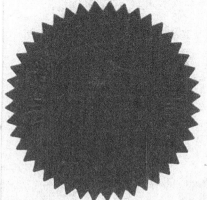

No. E 644

# Joint Nursing and Midwives Council for Northern Ireland.

*(12 and 13 Geo. V. Ch. 10.)*

**This is to Certify** that

Harriet May Thompson

was on the undermentioned date admitted by examination to the **Supplementary Part** of the Register maintained by the Joint Nursing and Midwives Council for Northern Ireland, containing the names of Nurses trained in the Nursing of persons suffering from Infectious Diseases; and that she is entitled in pursuance of the Joint Nursing and Midwives Council Act (Northern Ireland), 1922, to take and use the title of "Registered Fever Nurse."

Dated this *twenty-second*

day of *October*, 1947.

*James Boyd.*
Chairman.

*M. C. Poole*
Registrar.

4.8 Joint Nursing and Midwives Council for Northern Ireland, 1947: Harriet May Thompson.

No. 382

# Kings Cross Hospital
### for Infectious Diseases
## Dundee

## We hereby Certify

That        *Elma Petrie*

has been trained in the wards of this Hospital for the full term of three years from    *1.1.52* to    *1.1.55*        and has acquitted herself satisfactorily.    She has attended courses of instruction and passed an examination on the following subjects.

| | |
|---|---|
| Anatomy & Physiology | Infectious Diseases |
| Hygiene | Medical and Surgical Nursing |
| Dietetics and Invalid Cookery | Practical Nursing. |

Signed this *31st* day of *December, 1954.*

*Gladys E. Merritt,* R.G.N., R.F.N. Reg Tutor Matron

*William L. Januim.* M.D., D.P.H.        Medical Superintendent.

4.9 King's Cross Hospital for Infectious Diseases, Dundee, 1955: Elma Petrie.

4.10 Dublin Fever Hospital, 1959: Bridget Mary Geraghty.

# Bibliography

The place of publication is London, unless stated otherwise.

Abel-Smith, B. (1960) *A History of the Nursing Profession*, Heinemann.

Abel-Smith, B. (1964) *The Hospitals 1800–1948: A Study in Social Administration in England and Wales*, Heinemann.

Allan, P. and Jolley, M. (eds) *Nursing, Midwifery and Health Visiting since 1900*, Faber & Faber.

Anderson, M. (ed.) (1996) *British Population History: From the Black Death to the Present Day*, Cambridge: Cambridge University Press.

Aycliffe, G. A. and English, M. P. (2003) *Hospital Infection from Miasmas to MRSA*, Cambridge: Cambridge University Press.

Ayers, G. M. (1971) *England's First State Hospitals and the Metropolitan Asylums Board 1867–1930*, Wellcome Institute of the History of Medicine.

Baly, M. E. (1980) *Nursing and Social Change* (2nd edn), Heinemann.

Baly, M. E. (1995) *Nursing and Social Change* (3rd edn), Routledge.

Baly, M. (ed.) (1997) *As Miss Nightingale Said . . . Florence Nightingale through her Sayings – A Victorian Perspective* (2nd edn), Baillière Tindall, in association with the Royal College of Nursing.

Behlmer, G. K. (1982) *Child Abuse and Moral Reform in England, 1870–1908*, Stanford, CA: Stanford University Press.

Bell, E. M. (1962) *Josephine Butler: Flame of Fire*, Constable.

Bendall, E. R. D. and Raybould, E. (1969) *A History of the General Nursing Council for England and Wales 1919–1969*, Lewis.

*Black's Medical Dictionary*, 1916.

Brown, K. (2004). *Penicillin Man. Alexander Fleming and the Antibiotic Revolution*, Stroud, Sutton.

Buchan, W. (1824[1769]) *Domestic Medicine: A Treatise on the Prevention and Cure of Diseases by Regimen and Simple Medicines*, Bumpus.

Burdett, H. C. (1893) *Hospitals and Asylums of the World: Their Origin, History, Construction, Administration, Management, and Legislation* [in 4 vols], *and the Portfolio of Plans*, Scientific.

Burdett, H. C. (ed.) (1927) *How to become a Nurse: A Complete Guide to Training in the Profession of Nursing* (11th edn), Scientific.

*Burdett's Hospitals and Charities*.

Burne, J. (1996) *Dartford's Capital River: Paddle Steamers, Personalities and Smallpox Boats*, Buckingham: Baron.

Cashman, B. (1988) *Private Charity and the Public Purse: The Development of Bedford General Hospital 1794–1988*, Bedford: North Bedfordshire Health Authority.

Clark-Kennedy, A. E. (1965) *Edith Cavell, Pioneer and Patriot*, Faber & Faber.

Clarkson, L. A. and Crawford, M. E. (2001) *Food and Nutrition in Ireland 1800–1920*, New York: Oxford University Press.

Clay, R. M. (1909) *The Medieval Hospitals of England*, Methuen.

Coleman, D. and Salt, J. (1992) *The British Population: Patterns, Trends, and Processes*, Oxford: Oxford University Press.

Cook, C. and Stevenson, J. (1988) *The Longman Handbook of Modern British History 1714–1987* (2nd edn), Longman.

Creighton, C. (1891, 1894) *A History of Epidemics in Britain* (2 vols), vol. 1, *A History of Epidemics in Britain from AD 664 to the Extinction of the Plague*; vol. 2, *From the Extinction of the Plague to the Present Time*, Cambridge: Cambridge University Press.

Currie, M. R. (1982) *Hospitals in Luton and Dunstable: An Illustrated History*, Hitchin: Advance Offset.

Daunton, C. (ed.) (1990) *Edith Cavell: Her Life and her Art*, Royal London Hospital.

Davies, C. (ed.) (1980) *Rewriting Nursing History*, Croom Helm.

Dingwall, H. M. (2003) *A History of Scottish Medicine: Themes and Influences*, Edinburgh: Edinburgh University Press.

Dingwall, R., Rafferty, A.M. and Webster, C. (1988) *An Introduction to the Social History of Nursing*, Routledge.

Donahue, P. M. (1996) *Nursing, the Finest Art: An Illustrated History*, St Louis, MO: Mosby.

Donnelly, J. S. Jr (2001) *The Great Irish Potato Famine*, Stroud: Sutton.

Dundas, G. H. G. (1924) *Text-book for Fever Nurses*, Edinburgh: Bryce.

Emrys-Roberts, M. (1991) *The Cottage Hospitals 1859–1990*, Motcombe, Dorset: Tern.

Engels, F. (1969[1845]) *The Condition of the Working Class in England from Personal Observation and Authentic Sources*, Panther.

Eyler, J. M. (1997) *Sir Arthur Newsholme and State Medicine, 1885–1935*, Cambridge: Cambridge University Press.

Foucault, M. (1991[1975]) *Discipline and Punish: The Birth of the Prison*, trans. A. M. Sheridan, Penguin.

Foucault, M. (2003[1963]) *The Birth of the Clinic: An Archaeology of Medical Perception*, trans. A. M. Sheridan, Routledge Classics.

Frazer, W. M. (1950) *A History of English Public Health, 1834–1939*, Baillière, Tindall & Cox.

Gardiner, J. and Wenborn, N. (eds) (1995) *The History Today Companion to British History*, Collins & Brown.

Goffman, E. (1991[1961]) *Asylums: Essays on the Social Situation of Mental Patients and other Inmates*, Penguin.

Gould, T. (1995) *A Summer Plague: Polio and its Survivors*, New Haven, CT: Yale University Press.

Granshaw, L. and Porter, R. (eds) (1990) *The Hospital in History*, Routledge.

Gray, J. A. (1999) *The Edinburgh City Hospital*, East Lothian: Tuckwell Press.

Halsey, A. H. (ed.) (1972) *Trends in British Society since 1900: A Guide to the Changing Social Structure of Britain*, Macmillan.

Halsey, A. H. (ed.) (1988) *British Social Trends since 1900: A Guide to the Changing Social Structure of Britain* (2nd edn), Macmillan.

Hardy, A. (1993) *The Epidemic Streets: Infectious Disease and the Rise of Preventive Medicine 1856–1900*, Oxford: Clarendon Press.

Hardy, A. (2001) *Health and Medicine in Britain since 1860*, Basingstoke: Palgrave.

Illich, I. (1990[1976]) *Limits to Medicine: Medical Nemesis – the Expropriation of Health*, Penguin.

Laidlaw, E. F. (1990) *The Story of the Royal National Hospital, Ventnor*, Newport, Isle of Wight: Crossprint (private publication by the author).

Lane, J. (2000) *The Making of the English Patient: A Guide to Sources for the Social History of Medicine*, Stroud: Sutton.

Lane, J. (2001) *A Social History of Medicine: Health, Healing and Disease in England, 1750–1950*, Routledge.

Lewis, J. (1986) *What Price Community Medicine? The Philosophy, Practice and Politics of Public Health since 1919*, Brighton: Wheatsheaf.

Linnell, C. D. (ed.) (1999[1949]) *Historical Carlton through the Diary of Benjamin Rogers, Rector of Carlton, 1720–1771*, Carlton and Chellington Historical Society.

McCleary, G. F. (1935) *The Maternity and Child Welfare Movement*, King.

Macdonald, L. (1993) *The Roses of No Man's Land*, Penguin.

McGann, S. (1992) *The Battle of the Nurses: A Study of Eight Women who Influenced the Development of Professional Nursing, 1880–1930*, Scutari Press.

McKenzie, P. (2000) *Fevers, Family and Friends: A Memoir*, University of Glasgow, Wellcome Unit for the History of Medicine.

McKeown, T. and Lowe, C. R. (1974) *An Introduction to Social Medicine* (2nd edn), Oxford: Blackwell Scientific.

McLachlan, G. (ed.) (1987) *Improving the Common Weal: Aspects of the Scottish Health Service, 1900–1984*, Edinburgh: Edinburgh University Press for the Nuffield Provincial Hospital Trust.

Maclean, H. (1932) *Nursing in New Zealand: History and Reminiscences*, Wellington, NZ: Tolan.

Mangold, T. and Goldberg, A. (1999) *Plague Wars: A True Story of Biological Warfare*, Macmillan.

Merry, E. J. and Irven, I. D. (1960) *District Nursing: A Handbook for District Nurses and for All Concerned in the Administration of a District Nursing Service*, Baillière, Tindall & Cox.

Monk, A. S. (1978) *Fairfield Hospital: A Short History of the Hospital 1860–1960*, Hitchin: Fairfield Hospital.

Morten, H. (n.d.[1899]) *How to Become a Nurse and How to Succeed*, Scientific.

Newman, G. (1906) *Infant Mortality: A Social Problem*, Methuen.

Nightingale, F. (1969[1860]) *Notes on Nursing: What It is, and What It is Not*, New York: Dover.

Parish, H. J. (1965) *A History of Immunization*, Edinburgh: Livingstone.

Parker, E. R. and Collins, S. M. (1998) *Learning to Care: A History of Nursing and Midwifery Education at the Royal London Hospital, 1740–1993*, Royal London Hospital Archives and Museum.

Pearce, E. (1940) *Fevers and Fever Nursing* (4th edn), Faber & Faber.

Pelling, M. (1978) *Cholera, Fever and English Medicine*, Oxford: Oxford University Press.

Perks, R. (1992) *Oral History: Talking about the Past*, Historical Association.

Pinker, R. (1966) *English Hospital Statistics 1861–1938*, Heinemann.

Porter, R. (1997) *The Greatest Benefit to Mankind: A Medical History of Humanity from Antiquity to the Present*, HarperCollins.

Porter, R. and Wear, A. (1987) *Problems and Methods in the History of Medicine*, Croom Helm.

Prochaska, F. (1988) *The Voluntary Impulse: Philanthropy in Modern Britain*, Faber & Faber.

Rackstraw, M. (ed.) (n.d.[1926]) *A Social Survey of the City of Edinburgh*, Edinburgh: Oliver & Boyd for the Council of Social Service.

Rafferty, A.M. (1996) *The Politics of Nursing Knowledge*, London: Routledge.

Rafferty, A.M., Robinson, J. and Elkan, R. (eds) (1997) *Nursing History and the Politics of Welfare*, Routledge.

Ranger, T. and Slack, P. (eds) (1992) *Epidemics and Ideas: Essays on the Historical Perception of Pestilence*, Cambridge: Cambridge University Press.

Richardson, H. (ed.) (1998) *English Hospitals 1660–1948: A Survey of their Architecture and Design*, Swindon: Royal Commission on the Historical Monuments of England.

Richardson, R. (1989) *Death, Dissection and the Destitute*, Penguin.

Riddell, M. S. (n.d.[1914]) *Lectures to Nurses: Being a Complete Series of Lectures to Probationary Nurses in their First, Second and Third Year of Training*, Scientific.

Risse, G. B. (1999) *Mending Bodies, Saving Souls: A History of Hospitals*, New York: Oxford University Press.

Robins, J. (2000) *Nursing and Midwifery in Ireland in the Twentieth Century: Fifty Years of An Bord Altranais (The Nursing Board), 1950–2000*, Dublin: An Bord Altranais.

Rosenberg, C. E. (1992) *Explaining Epidemics and other Studies in the History of Medicine*, Cambridge: Cambridge University Press.

Ryder, R. (1975) *Edith Cavell*, Hamish Hamilton.

Scanlan, P. (1991) *The Irish Nurse – A Study of Nursing in Ireland: History and Education, 1718–1981*, Co. Leitrim, Northern Ireland: Drumlin.

Schorr, T. M. and Kennedy, M. S. (1999) *100 Years of American Nursing: Celebrating a Century of Caring*, Philadelphia, PA: Lippincott.

Searle, C. (1965) *The History of the Development of Nursing in South Africa 1652–1960 (A Socio-Historical Survey)*, Cape Town: Struik.

Selby-Green, J. (1990) *The History of the Radcliffe Infirmary*, Banbury: Image Publications.

Sherwood, T. (1641) *The Charitable Pestmaster or the Cure of the Plague*, John Francklin.

Smiles, S. (1860[1859]) *Self-help; with Illustrations of Character and Conduct*, John Murray.

Smith, F. B. (1979) *The People's Health 1830–1910*, New York: Holmes & Meier.

Smith, J. P. (1989) *Virginia Henderson: The First Ninety Years*, Scutari.

Sworder, H. (1893) *Popular Information Concerning Infectious Diseases*, Henry Renshaw.

Taylor, J. (1991) *Hospital and Asylum Architecture in England 1840–1914: Building for Health Care*, Mansell.

Thompson, F. M. L. (ed.) (1990) *The Cambridge Social History of Britain 1750–1950* (3 vols), vol. 2, *People and their Environment*, Cambridge: Cambridge University Press.

Thompson, J. I. (n.d.) *Belvoir Park Hospital: Fever 1840s-1986*, Belfast (private publication).

Thompson, P. (1988) *The Voice of the Past: Oral History* (2nd edn), Oxford: Oxford University Press.

Underwood, A. (1974) *'Home Rule for Ampthill': A Summary of the Town's Government through the Urban District Council and its Antecedents*, Ampthill Urban District Council.

Watson, J. M. (1939) *Aids to Fever Nursing*, Baillière, Tindall & Cox.

Watson, J. M. (1945) *Aids to Fevers for Nurses* (2nd edn), Baillière, Tindall & Cox.

Webster, C. (1988) *The Health Services since the War*, vol. 1, *Problems of Health Care: The NHS before 1957*, HMSO.

Weeks, J. (1989) *Sex, Politics and Society: The Regulation of Sexuality since 1800* (2nd edn), Longman.

Wesley, J. (1960[1747]) *Primitive Physic or An Easy and Natural Method of Curing most Diseases*, Epworth Press.

Whitteridge, G. and Stokes, V. (1961) *A Brief History of the Hospital of Saint Bartholomew*, Governors of the Hospital of Saint Bartholomew.

Wohl, A. S. (1983) *Endangered Lives: Public Health in Victorian Britain*, Dent.

Woodforde, J. (1978) *The Diary of a Country Parson (1758–1802)*, passages selected and edited by J. Beresford, Oxford: Oxford University Press.

Woods, R. and Woodward, J. (eds) (1984) *Urban Disease and Mortality in Nineteenth Century England*, Batsford.

Woodward, J. (1974) *To Do the Sick No Harm: A Study of the British Voluntary Hospital System to 1875*, Routledge & Kegan Paul.

Woolacott, F. J. (1906) *Lectures upon the Nursing of Infectious Diseases*, Scientific Press.

Zimmerman, B. E. and Zimmerman, D. J. (2003) *Killer Germs: Microbes and Diseases that Threaten Humanity*, Chicago: Contemporary Books.

# Index

Printed and bound by CPI Group (UK) Ltd, Croydon, CR0 4YY

01/11/2024

01782626-0012